The Future Of Sleep

The Future Of Sleep

Catherine Ball

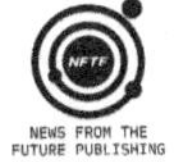

NEWS FROM THE
FUTURE PUBLISHING

ISBN Paperback: 978-1-7643013-0-5

ISBN EBook: 978-1-7643013-1-2

Publisher: News From The Future Publishing

Cover Design: Jeremy Fay

First Edition: Feb, 2026

CONTENTS

| VI | –

Prologue

For those seeking better sleep.

I truly hope this is a useful compass, map, and field guide.

Important Note: I am not a medically trained doctor, I am a scientist and technologist. If you are having any concerns about your health or your sleep, please do see your GP/personal doctor about it.

This book is for education and entertainment only and is not intended to be medical advice so don't take it as such.

“ I have spread my dreams under your feet. ”

Tread softly because you tread on my dreams.

W. B. YEATS

Dedication

This book is dedicated to the memory of Myra Juliet Farrell.

In the quiet suburbs of Australia, during the early twentieth century, lived a woman named Myra Juliet Farrell. To her neighbours she was an eccentric character, but to the patent office she was a veritable force of nature. Myra was not a trained engineer; she was a composer and an artist who happened to possess a rather unusual manufacturing process. She did not toil over blueprints at a drafting table or spend late nights tinkering in a shed, instead, when Myra faced a mechanical problem she could not solve, she simply went to bed and fell asleep.

Myra realised early in life that her subconscious mind was a far better engineer than her waking one and if she needed to invent a device, she would focus on the problem intensely before retiring for the night, essentially briefing her sleeping brain on the task at hand. One of her most famous successes involved the labour of sewing buttons. Frustrated by the needle and thread, she took the problem to sleep and woke up with the design for the *stitchless press stud*. She sketched the vision on her bedside table, and the invention became a commercial hit that allowed fasteners to be attached mechanically rather than sewn by hand.

Her nocturnal workshop produced an incredible range of innovations. Myra secured more than two dozen patents in her lifetime, ranging from a mechanical fruit picker that could harvest high branches without bruising the skin to the folding pram hood that became a standard design for baby carriages. She famously told a newspaper reporter in 1915 that she often went to bed early because she had work to do. While the rest of Australia saw sleep as a time of inactivity, Myra saw it as her second shift, trusting that the solution would arrive in the theatre of her dreams.

Myra Juliet Farrell is the patron saint of this book because she represents the shift from viewing sleep as a biological tax to viewing it as a biological tool. She understood instinctively what neuroscientists are only now beginning to prove, which is that the sleeping brain is not offline. It is busy connecting disparate ideas, running simulations, and testing structural integrity in a way the conscious mind cannot. She did not sleep to escape her problems; she slept to solve them. Legend.

Introduction: Reclaiming the Night

Sleep is the single most effective thing we can do to reset our brain and body health each day. It is the Swiss Army knife of health.

MATTHEW WALKER, WHY WE SLEEP

Why do we sleep?

It is a question that science still lacks a complete and singular answer for, but ultimately sleep is a defining feature of being human. We often treat sleep as a passive state, a period of nothingness that happens between the productive parts of our lives. Evolutionarily speaking, sleep is a multi-species phenomenon and has proved too useful to delete, i.e. if we could survive without it, we would have evolved to do so by now. Instead, we carry an undeniable and built-in night shift that persists regardless of our social obligations, our work rosters, or the blue light emanating from our bedside tables and smart devices.

Technically, we are never truly off during the night. While we sleep, our bodies and brains are actually incredibly active. Filing memories, resetting the immune system, and tuning the hormonal balance are just the beginning of the brain's nocturnal workload. Meanwhile, the heart, liver, gut, and kidneys take their own night shifts, performing essential maintenance that cannot be conducted while we are upright and alert.

When scientists have searched for clues as to a single, definitive reason for sleep in humans, they simply haven't found one; they have found quite a few. Sleep helps consolidate knowledge and clears waste from the brain through what we now understand as the glymphatic system. It recharges immune cells and ensures our emotional regulation remains intact for the coming day. We have many important reasons why we need to protect it, yet it is the first thing that suffers when we are running mad in our busy lives.

The Lost History of Rest and Getting Knocked Up

How we sleep has changed radically over the last few centuries, and we have not always slept the way we currently do. In parts of pre-industrial Europe, there was a common practice of sleeping in two sessions also called biphasic sleep; a veritable split shift of sleep. Historians call this a first sleep and a second sleep and it was even written about by the likes of Chaucer in his stories, as well as other famous ballads and poems. There was even medical advice in the 15th century to sleep on the right hand side for the first sleep and the left hand side for the second sleep to aid digestion (though that should probably be the other way round when you think about anatomy).

The stretch of wakefulness in the middle of the night was apparently a period of high social and personal utility, and for some people the opportunity for crime and bad behaviour. It was more typically used for chores, reading, sex, and prayer or even a quiet chat with your family or neighbours. Do you wake up at 1am and stay awake 'til 3am?

Talk about waking up; it wasn't until 1787 that the alarm clock was actually invented by an American chap called Levi Hutchins who wanted to wake up every day at 4am, before sunrise. He was a clock maker but never made the alarm variety for anyone else to use. The first patented mechanical alarm clock was registered by Frenchman Antoine Redier in 1847. Who would have thought that horology from centuries ago would be such a disruptive force in the modern bedroom? I used to use alarm clocks, now I have small children that act as personal 'knocker-uppers' for me on a daily basis. People in the UK were paid in the industrial revolution right up to the 1970s to run around waking people up for work by knocking (or using a pea shooter) on their window or door, charging for the service to 'knock you up'. Now that expression means something else entirely.

The biggest industrial disruption to sleep came not from sound or being knocked up, but from light! Gaslight was the first method used to stretch the evenings into productivity, starting in the early 1800s. This changed how people worked in offices and factories, and how late shops and taverns stayed open. As we moved to electric light, there was a scaling of this night-lighting of our lives via a cheaper, brighter, and safer mechanism, even moving indoors. Edison (and his light bulb) didn't only sell the idea of increased recreation; he sold a longer day. People making money off the working class recognised this as a golden opportunity to make themselves richer and more successful.

In the mid-2020s, it must be acknowledged that we are living in a rather tired century, and cheap electricity is partly to blame. Electric light does two direct things that matter for sleep. It allows us to keep doing things after dark and thereby increases the work and brain use outside of normal hours. It also changes the biology of the night directly by removing our connection to sunset and sunrise. Even ordinary room light in the evening suppresses melatonin and shortens the internal sense of night. By shortening the sense of night, we suddenly find ourselves in a bit of a paradox; trying to fall asleep quickly while not allowing the time the brain chemistry needs to enable us to fall asleep. Don't even start about daylight savings time in the summer in Australia and trying to get my kids to sleep.

We make it hard for ourselves to drift off to sleep early enough most nights, and this is all without any doom scrolling on handheld screens involved in the equation. It isn't the effect of one harsh bulb; it is the glow of the whole home. As parents or carers, we can easily find ourselves trapped in an ouroboros of sleep deprivation. We stay up late just to get well-needed alone time, a phenomenon known as revenge bedtime procrastination, which actually creates a larger sleep deficit. Sometimes as parents of young children it feels like we just cannot win. The biggest reward we can give ourselves is a chance for more rest, not less. We need to stop equating binge watching a crappy series as a reward, it is nothing more than cheap dopamine overload; chewing gum for the brain.

The Sleep Economy: From Tracking to Prediction

One of the main questions we ask ourselves about sleep is purely quantitative: 'how many hours is enough'? The answer is hotly debated and not an easy one (nor am I qualified to answer). The general consensus is that sleep quantity is not proportional to sleep quality. Sleep requirements change for us individually based on age, stage of life, and gender. Different studies have typically averaged the numbers to over 6 hours sleep required per night, with women needing more like between 8-10 hours. This is especially important during perimenopause and menopause, stages of life that have been historically ignored in sleep literature (and also in some best-selling books on sleep, thanks to mostly male authors getting the breaks in this area).

I am not a sleep specialist by profession, so I turn to the academic literature and the recent books on sleep and the ecosystem of research responses. As a mother with a newborn baby a few years ago, if someone even dared to suggest that I needed 8 hours, or to 'sleep when the baby sleeps' they would have been given a withering look at the very least. Everyone has an opinion about sleep and most aren't afraid to share it. However, as we personalise the 'internet of bodies' for our wearables to tell us more about our sleep quantity and give us quality scores, we are now swimming in marketing and potentially erroneous information. They call it the sleep economy for a reason; someone, somewhere, wants to make a lot of money from it (read: make a lot of money from *you*).

We are currently entering a new phase of this economy. Let's call it Sleep 3.0. In the previous decade, we were obsessed with tracking. We wore watches that told us we slept poorly, offering a score out of 100 that often served only to increase our anxiety: a condition clinicians now call 'orthosomnia'. But 2026 marks the shift from simple tracking to predictive diagnostics. We are seeing the rise of foundation models like SleepFM, developed by leading researchers at Stanford University, to do more than just count hours. These models use artificial intelligence to analyse thousands of hours of physiological data to identify the fingerprints of disease.

This technology does not just tell you that you tossed and turned; it identifies subtle asynchronies between your heart rate and your brain waves. These patterns can predict the risk of over 130 health conditions, including cardiovascular disease, Parkinson's, and dementia, years before clinical symptoms appear. This is the silent miracle of mathematics and AI: turning the bedroom from a place of passive rest into a preventative health clinic. It allows us to move from the quantified self to the qualified self, where data is used to support our biology rather than grade or rank it.

Light is not the only thing that has changed in recent decades. Work schedules and expectations have often been more disrespectful of our internal clocks than the LEDs we bathe ourselves in. Many of us live, work, and travel within schedules that do not respect our internal biological rhythms. The gap between our biological night and our social timetable has a formal name: social jetlag. You go to sleep and wake one way on workdays and then slide into something else on the weekends, desperate to catch up on a deficit you can't actually ever biologically refill.

The humanoid robotic revolution is upon us and will be scaled up by the end of this decade, but it has not yet (at the time of writing) removed the need for many human beings to do shift work. The average is about one in 10 workers must do nights.

Healthcare, logistics, hospitality, newsrooms, policing, and emergency services all run on bodies and minds that must stay awake and be able to make good decisions just when biology wants to sleep. There is a playbook for safer shifts to help protect our brains and bodies in ever increasing multimodal stressors that come alongside a messed up circadian rhythm, but we aren't ever taught about it in schools or by the health systems around us.

The Sleep Gap and Environmental Assault

How is our sleep being attacked while we don't even notice it anymore? I think it's akin to the frog in boiling water scenario. Areas we can review right now include the state of housing, heat in hotter cities, noise from cars and neighbours, and finally screens and wearables. Climate change is making our urban spaces hotter, and the lack of trees is adding to the heat island effect. As heat lingers into the night more often, it steals sleep by delaying the onset of and then also fragmenting the second half of the night.

Is a geographically related socio-economic sleep gap upon us? Older adults and people in lower income countries or socio-economic areas of western cities bear the burden harder. We are constantly told to eat the way our grandparents ate but I haven't started hearing yet the conversations around recommending that we sleep the way our grandparents slept. A midday nanna nap does not solve a chronic sleep deficit, though it may generate some alpha brain waves and allow a refresh. Just closing your eyes can change the way the brain processes information and give a refreshing effect despite you not actually falling asleep.

There is a clear demarcation when it comes to good sleep between those that can shape their nights and those that cannot. Is good quality sleep another indicator of privilege? If so, can technology be used to help democratise access to good quality rest? Ironically, technology is usually the target for blame. Since the advent of the very first iPhone in the year 2007, screens have become the prolific symbol of our era. It is simple to talk about light from a bright phone right next to your eyes delaying brain chemistry, but we must understand that behaviour beats technology. Put the device down, dim the room lights, and pick up a wind down habit.

We must also confront the gender data gap in sleep. For too long, medical research has treated the male body as the default, ignoring the distinct biological realities of half the population. This book gives space to the idea of motherhood and the transition into midlife, particularly menopause. Many of the big bestselling books on sleep don't even have the word menopause mentioned once; I intend to fix that in the one way I can, by including it in this work. We will look at how thermal technologies, smart mattresses and cooling wearables, are finally addressing the hot flashes and night sweats that disrupt the sleep of millions of women, treating these symptoms as addressable physiology rather than something to be endured in silence.

A Techno-Optimist's Field Guide

This book is a playbook and a field guide. We are going to walk through where technology is right now in the 2020s, where it's coming from, and how you can plan to have a tech-enabled better night of rest. I am a scientist and a techno-optimist, so you'll find that I've been looking for solutions here rather than focusing on the problems. We will start with the sensors on bodies and beds and move through artificial intelligence as a potential copilot. We will look at how the bedroom is becoming a clinic and what technologies now work at home.

I will really focus about owning the night in a world that wants to rent it back to you. We need to be careful about what we are handing over in order to access these dreamlike technologies. The "Internet of You" is growing, with sensors moving from our wrists to our ears and earlobes, and even under our skin, and all that data is going somewhere. We must ensure that privacy and dignity is built into these systems by design. We do not want an AI assistant selling us products while we are unconscious. Part of owning the night is demanding that our data remains ours, stored locally or shared only with explicit, revocable consent.

The sleep economy is estimated to reach a value of nearly 100 billion US dollars globally by the end of this decade, spanning across wearables, smart mattresses, and digital therapeutics. Yet, the most valuable part of this economy is not the gadgets you buy, but the time you reclaim. We must address the sleep gap, ensuring that the benefits of this revolution are not reserved only for those with the deepest pockets. From adolescent school starts to the right to disconnect from work, the future of sleep is as much about policy and culture as it is about silicon and code.

In the chapters that follow, we will dissect the hype, debunk the myths, and look closely at the harms that can arise when technology is implemented without ethical guardrails. We will look at engineering dreams and resting when the stakes are high, whether you are a global executive or a parent on the midnight shift. Ultimately, this book is about agency. It is about understanding the switches for calm that already exist in your body, like the vagus nerve and the breath, and using technology to amplify them, not replace them.

It is time to treat sleep as the personalised health and economic engine it has always been.

The night belongs to you; now let's technologically augment it, together.

1

The Next Sleep Revolution

WILLIAM SHAKESPEARE

The Vanishing Night

The night has become a design space, a data collection cru-cible, and a personal laboratory. It is a profound shift for a species that, for ninety-nine per cent of its history, viewed the time after sunset as a domain defined strictly by what was absent. For millennia, the human experience of the night was characterised by the absence of labour, the absence of travel, and, most critically, the absence of artificial light. When the sun dipped below the horizon, biology took the cue. The ambient temperature dropped, the visual world faded into greyscale, and the human body slipped into a mode of preservation and recovery. The night belonged to the stars, to the nocturnal hunters, and to the quiet, communal safety of the group huddled around a fire. It was a time for storytelling, for physical closeness, and eventually, for a profound and un-monitored silence.

That version of the night is effectively extinct. We have replaced the canopy of stars with a ceiling of standby lights. If you wake up in a modern bedroom at 3am and look around, you are unlikely to see true darkness. Instead, you are met with the blinking red eye of a smoke detector, the soft white glow of a Wi-Fi router, the green charge indicator on a laptop, and the blue digits of a clock. We have traded the infinite depth of the night sky for the blinking and unblinking constellations of our smart devices. This is not merely an aesthetic change; it is a fundamental rewiring of the human experience. We have taken the one period of the day that was evolutionarily designed for disconnection and filled it with indicators of connectivity.

It was Thomas Edison's lab workers, and the advent of the electric light that truly broke the connection between the sun and our sleep. Edison did not just sell a light bulb; he sold the idea of a longer day. He marketed the concept of increased recreation, but more importantly for the industrialists of the time, he sold increased economic output. People making money off the working class recognised this as a golden opportunity to make themselves richer and more successful. The factory whistle replaced the rooster, and the electric bulb replaced the sun. We successfully engineered the night out of existence.

In the mid-2020s, we are living in the tired century that Edison helped create. Cheap electricity is partly to blame for our collective exhaustion. Electric light does two direct things that matter for sleep. First, it allows us to keep doing things after dark, thereby increasing work and brain use outside of normal physiological hours. We can answer emails at midnight, do laundry at 2am, and binge-watch television until dawn. I can even edit this book at 10pm.

Second, and more insidiously, it changes the biology of the night directly by removing our connection to sunset and sunrise. Even ordinary room light in the evening is bright enough to suppress the release of melatonin, the hormone that signals darkness to the body. By suppressing melatonin and maintaining alertness, we shorten our internal sense of night. We find ourselves in a paradox. We try to fall asleep quickly to maximise our limited rest time, while simultaneously denying ourselves the brain chemistry required to drift off. We make it hard for ourselves to sleep, and this is all without even factoring in the dopamine-fuelled doom scrolling on handheld screens that keeps us psychologically engaged when we should be winding down.

This shift has created a vacuum that technology is now rushing to fill. We have broken our sleep with technology, and now we are turning to more technology to fix it. This is the irony at the heart of the next sleep revolution. We are attempting to use the very tools that disrupted our circadian rhythms to re-pair them. We are fighting fire with data.

But this new revolution is different from the industrial one. It is not about conquering the night. It is about reclaiming it, but on very specific terms. We are entering a decade where the bedroom is no longer a neutral space. It is readable and programmable. We are seeing a tectonic shift from lab break-throughs to startup investments that land directly on our bed-side tables. Marketing gurus aim these devices squarely at the worried well. These are people who aren't sick but also have money and the desire to stay that way.

The goal for many is no longer just to rest, but to win at sleep-ing. We want the perfect score. We want the graph that proves we recovered. We want to engineer the perfect night because we feel so out of control during the day. The sleep economy has arisen to service this need. It is a multi-billion dollar indus-try built on the anxiety that we are doing sleep wrong. It in-cludes everything from the mattress you lie on to the ring on your finger, the pill you swallow, and the app that whispers stories to you.

Social jetlag is the price we pay for this misalignment. It is the gap between our biological night and our social timetable. You go to sleep and wake one way on workdays, constrained by the alarm clock, and then slide into a different pattern on the weekends, desperate to catch up on a deficit you can never actually refill. We experience parental jetlag, newborn jetlag, and overstressed jetlag. It seems that nothing about modern life actually respects our biological sleep needs, and neither do we.

So, we turn to the new tools. We invite the sensors in. We replace the stars with the status LED because we are looking for a compass. We want something to tell us that we are okay, or to tell us how to be better. The night has become crowded. Instead of the silence of our ancestors, we have the hum of the air purifier, the white noise machine, the vibration of the smart watch, and the silent, invisible polling of the radar sensor.

This is the reality of the next sleep revolution. It is not a return to the paleolithic sleep of our ancestors, where we might have dozed in thirty-minute bursts safe from predators.

We cannot go back to that. We are moving forward into a future where the night is technologically augmented. The question is no longer whether we should bring technology into the bedroom, as it is already there. The question is who owns that technology, who owns the data it generates, and whether it is actually helping us rest or just giving us one more thing to worry about in the dark.

We are standing at the threshold of a new era where the human body is fully integrated into the internet of things, even when it is unconscious. The challenge of this book, and of the coming decade, is to navigate this new landscape without losing the essential, restorative magic of sleep itself. We need to learn how to use these tools to support our biology rather than distract from it. We need to find a way to turn off the status LEDs, or at least tape over them, and find a version of the night that works for the modern human. The revolution is here, and it is wearing a wristband.

The Rise of the Sleep Economy

We have turned the most natural human function into a product line. If you walk through a modern department store or scroll through the health section of a digital marketplace, you will see the physical evidence of a massive cultural shift. What was once a simple biological necessity, free of charge and requiring no equipment other than a horizontal surface, has been repackaged as a premium lifestyle pursuit. Sleep is no longer something you just do. It is now something you (can) buy.

This commodification has birthed what industry analysts now call the sleep economy. It is a sprawling, multi-billion dollar ecosystem that services our collective exhaustion. In 2024, the global market for sleep technology devices alone was valued at over twenty billion US dollars, and aggressive forecasts suggest it could cross the one hundred billion dollar mark by the early 2030s. When you add in mattresses, pharmaceuticals, supplements, and sleep tourism, the total value swells to hundreds of billions. This is not a niche market for insomniacs anymore. It is a mainstream juggernaut that rivals the fitness industry in scale and ambition.

The fuel for this economic engine is a specific type of modern anxiety. Marketing departments have zeroed in on a demographic known to some as the worried well, and to others as the tech-centric longevity bros who created the 5am club. These are people who do not necessarily suffer from clinical sleep disorders like narcolepsy or severe sleep apnoea. Instead, they are the functional but fatigued millions who feel that they are underperforming. They are the professionals who believe that if they could just tweak their REM cycle efficiency by five per cent, they would finally get that promotion or write that novel. They are the parents who are terrified that their own sleep deprivation is trickling down to their children. They have disposable income, high standards for personal optimisation, and a nagging suspicion that they are doing sleep wrong.

For this group, sleep has moved from being a restorative pause to being a performance metric. We treat recovery like a competitive sport. The sleep economy sells the promise that with the right gear, you can hack your biology. You can buy a ring that tracks your heart rate variability to the millisecond. You can subscribe to an app that uses artificial intelligence to compose a lullaby specifically for your brainwaves. You can purchase a mattress that costs as much as a small car because it promises to lower your core body temperature by the exact degree required for deep sleep.

The shift is visible in where the money is flowing. Venture capital funding for sleep technology startups has surged, doubling in volume between 2017 and 2021. In 2024 and 2025 alone, millions of dollars were poured into companies developing everything from AI powered coaching platforms to headbands that use acoustic stimulation to induce drowsiness, or vagus nerve stimulators. Investors are betting big on the idea that we are willing to pay a monthly subscription for the privilege of resting. They are banking on sleep becoming a service rather than a right.

This financial boom has changed the texture of the bedroom. It is no longer just a room with a bed; it is a showroom for the latest innovations in the internet of bodies. We see the rise of the invisible interface, where technology recedes into the fabric of the room. The market for non-wearable devices, such as smart mattresses and bedside radar units that track breathing without touching the skin, is projected to grow rapidly as people tire of wearing plastic gadgets to bed. The goal is zero friction monitoring, where the act of being measured becomes as passive as the act of sleeping itself.

However, there is a shadow side to this commercialisation. As we flood the market with tools to measure and optimise sleep, we risk creating a new psychological disorder. Clinicians have coined the term orthosomnia to describe an unhealthy obsession with achieving perfect sleep data. It is a cruel irony. The person suffering from orthosomnia might wake up feeling refreshed, check their sleep score, see a low number, and immediately feel tired and anxious. The data overrides their own internal experience. The quest for the perfect night becomes the very thing that keeps them awake.

The sleep economy thrives on this insecurity. It needs you to feel that your natural sleep is insufficient so that it can sell you the solution. It tells you that your prehistoric biological rhythms are incompatible with the modern world, which is true, but then suggests that the answer is a digital patch rather than a lifestyle change. It focuses on individual optimisation because that is what can be packaged and sold. It is much harder to sell a product that fixes the structural causes of sleep loss, like shift work schedules, noise pollution, or economic stress. So instead, we get lavender infused pillows and smart eye masks with white noise.

We are also seeing a demographic shift in who is buying these products. While the twenty to thirty nine year old age group has historically dominated the market, the fastest growth is now expected among those aged forty to fifty nine. This generation is squeezed between caring for children and ageing parents, often at the peak of their careers, and facing the physiological changes of midlife. For them, sleep is the first casualty of a busy life, and they are willing to pay a premium to reclaim it. They are driving the demand for more sophisticated, medical grade devices that offer more than just a step count. They want clinical insights without the hospital visit.

This demand is pushing consumer technology companies to act more like medical device manufacturers. The line between a wellness gadget and a medical tool is blurring. We now have consumer watches with FDA clearance to detect sleep apnoea risk and rings that claim to predict illness days before symptoms appear. This medicalisation of consumer goods is a key pillar of the sleep economy. It validates the purchase. You are not just buying a toy; you are investing in your healthspan and longevity.

Yet, amidst all this commerce, the fundamental nature of sleep remains stubbornly resistant to market forces. You cannot bribe your way into a good night's sleep. You can buy the best bed in the world, but if your mind is racing with worry or your circadian rhythm is out of sync with the sun, you will still stare at the ceiling. The sleep economy is excellent at selling us the hardware of sleep, the stage and the props, but it struggles to deliver the performance itself.

The danger is that by framing sleep as a commodity, we make it an exclusive luxury. We create a sleep gap where the wealthy can afford the cooling mattresses, the soundproof windows, and the personalised microbiome coaching, while the rest of society makes do with noise and heat. We risk viewing sleep not as a universal human right, but as a premium upgrade available to those who can afford the subscription fee.

As we move deeper into this decade, the sleep economy will only grow more pervasive. It will integrate with our smart homes, our insurance plans, and our healthcare systems. It will offer us more data, more control, and more promises of restoration. But we must remain critical consumers. We must remember that for thousands of years, humans slept perfectly well without apps or algorithms. The challenge is to use these new tools to support our biology, not to replace it with a business model. We need to ensure that in buying back the night, we do not end up selling our dreams.

The Sensor Invasion

To understand why your bedroom is suddenly filling up with technology, you do not need a degree in somnology. You need to look at the history of computing. There is a famous observation in the world of technology known as Moore's Law (from the man himself, the late, great, Gordon Moore). It states, roughly speaking, that the number of transistors on a microchip doubles about every two years, while the cost of computers is halved. This relentless march of miniaturisation is what turned room sized mainframes into the smartphone in your pocket. But for a long time, this exponential growth in processing power was mostly concerned with calculation and communication. It was about sending emails faster or rendering better video games. It had very little to do with the biological rhythms of the human body.

That changed when the sensors caught up with the processors. For decades, measuring the human body was a heavy, expensive, and industrial process. If you wanted to know your heart rhythm, you went to a hospital and were hooked up to a machine the size of a washing machine cart. If you wanted to measure your sleep, you went to a polysomnography lab, had wires glued to your scalp, face, and chest, and tried to sleep while a technician watched you from the next room. It was accurate, but it was artificial. It was medicine, not life.

Then the sensors shrank. The same economic forces that drove Moore's Law began to apply to the components that measure the physical world. Accelerometers, which measure movement, became microscopic and cheap enough to put in a phone to tell it which way was up. Photodiodes and LEDs, which can measure blood flow by shining light through the skin, became small enough to fit on the back of a watch. Batteries became efficient enough to run these things for days without charging.

This was the spark for the sensor explosion. We moved from a world where biological data was scarce, expensive, and episodic to a world where it is abundant, cheap, and continuous. We are entering a decade where most simplified biological data will be captured, archived, analysed, and predicted to provide us with personalised and tailored advice. This is a profound democratisation of medical grade insight. It means that the tools for understanding human physiology have escaped the hospital and moved into the wild.

Consider the sheer variety of form factors now available. We have wearables on wrists, fingers, and chests. We have caps that look like old school swimming caps but read brain waves. We have sensors under the mattress, on the mattress, in the blanket, on the pillow, and woven into pyjamas. We even have strips of tape or paper that act as sensors. All these wearable technologies are measuring and recording information such as breathing, heart rate variability, pulse, skin temperature, and whether you snore.

The industry calls this the invisible interface. The goal is to make the technology disappear so that you forget you are wearing it. A ring is less intrusive than a watch. A mat under the mattress is less intrusive than a ring. A radar on the bedside table is less intrusive than a mat. The trend is inexorably moving towards zero friction sensing. We are rapidly approaching a point where the environment itself monitors you, and you do not have to do anything other than lie down.

This explosion is fuelled by money. There is a lot of dollar in this tectonic shift, from lab breakthroughs to startup investments to our living rooms and kitchens. Investors have realised that sleep is a third of the human experience that has been largely unmonitored and unmonetised. If you can capture the data of the night, you own a massive slice of the human health picture.

The convergence of disparate arenas is what makes this moment unique. For the rest of this decade, we will see a huge amount of money being thrown at the intersection of sleep and emerging technology. Sensors and wireless chips have become small and cheap and easy to make. Artificial intelligence has learned enough about physiology in the last few years to be useful finally outside the hospital. At the same time, standards bodies globally have given us consistent ways to measure biological effective light, and regulators have started treating your sleep data as health information.

Put all these elements together and you have the perfect conditions for a revolution. It is no longer just about counting steps or measuring calories. It is about peering inside the autonomic nervous system. It is about using heart rate variability to gauge stress and recovery. It is about tracking the minute fluctuations in skin temperature that might signal the onset of an illness or a hormonal shift.

But there is a catch. This explosion of sensors has created a noisy marketplace. Not every sensor is created equal. A clinical grade pulse oximeter in a hospital is calibrated and regulated. A twenty dollar smart watch from a discount website is not. Yet they both produce a number on a screen that looks authoritative. We are swimming in data, but we are not always swimming in truth.

There is also the question of what we are actually measuring. Most consumer wearables do not yet diagnose diseases, but they are much better than they used to be at gathering data and sharing it with medical providers. In the pandemic, pulse and oxygen levels were being monitored via wearables at home to assist people who were unwell with COVID 19 without overwhelming the hospitals. This proved the utility of remote monitoring at scale. It showed that cheap sensors could provide a safety net.

However, the leap from useful trend data to medical diagnosis is a dangerous one to make without guidance. Smart wearables can estimate total sleep time and even attempt sleep staging with mixed accuracy when compared against the full polysomnography in a lab. This matters because the quality of rest and sleep timing even without perfect staging are incredibly useful baselines for adjusting your behaviour. But if the sensor says you got zero deep sleep and you panic, the sensor has done you a disservice.

Despite the risks, the trajectory is clear. The sensors will get smaller, cheaper, and more accurate. They will move from the outside of the body to the inside. We are already seeing the early days of ingestible sensors and implantable devices for sleep apnoea. The line between technology and biology is blurring.

The sensor explosion is not just about gadgets. It is about a fundamental change in our relationship with our own bodies. We used to listen to our bodies by feeling. We felt tired. We felt energetic. We felt wired. Now, we check our bodies. We look at the dashboard. We outsource our interoception to a silicon chip. This is the new reality of the next sleep revolution. We are the most measured humans in history. The question remains whether all this measurement is actually making us any better at sleeping, or if we are just watching ourselves toss and turn in high definition.

The Programmable Sanctuary

We tend to think of the bedroom as a static box. It has four walls, a ceiling, a floor, and a window. You put furniture in it, you paint the walls a colour you like, and then you leave it alone. The physics of the room, meaning the light, the temperature, the air composition, and the soundscape, are largely treated as fixed attributes of the house or the neighbourhood.

If you live on a busy street, your room is loud. If you live in a hot climate without air conditioning, your room is hot. We adapt ourselves to the room. We wear earplugs. We kick off the covers. We suffer through the stuffiness.

The next sleep revolution flips this dynamic on its head. It proposes that the bedroom should adapt to us. We are moving from the era of the static bedroom to the era of the programmable sanctuary. In this new paradigm, the room is a machine, and sleep is the function it is designed to optimise. This is not about interior design or feng shui. It is about environmental engineering applied to the domestic sphere.

The first and most critical variable in this programmable environment is light. For years, lighting designers measured light the way photographers do. They focused on lux and lumens, metrics that describe how bright a surface looks to the human eye. But biology cares about a different signal. Our eyes contain intrinsically photosensitive retinal ganglion cells that have nothing to do with vision and everything to do with time. These cells detect specific wavelengths of blue rich light and send signals directly to the master clock in the brain, the suprachiasmatic nucleus.

We now have a new international standard for measuring this biological signal, known as melanopic equivalent daylight illuminance. This sounds deeply technical, but its implication is practical and profound. It means we can now rate a light bulb not just by how it looks, but by how it affects your hormones. We are moving towards a world where your bedroom lights will automatically shift their spectrum and intensity to match the time of day. In the morning, they will deliver a high dose of melanopic light to suppress melatonin and wake you up. In the evening, they will drop to zero melanopic impact, allowing the hormone of darkness to rise, even if the room is still illuminated enough to read a book. Expect to see lamps, blinds, and operating systems that present these numbers as routinely as we see watts or volts. The programmable room will handle this choreography for you. You will not notice the algorithm. You will just notice that you feel sleepy at the right time.

The second lever in the programmable environment is temperature. If you have ever been one of those people who has thrown a leg out of the doona/duvet at 3am, you already know that temperature is the steering wheel of sleep biology. To fall asleep, your core body temperature needs to drop by about one degree Celsius. To stay asleep, it needs to stay low. The body sheds heat through the skin of the hands and feet to make this happen.

The static bedroom fights this process. Most mattresses are made of foam, which is excellent for comfort but terrible for heat regulation. It acts as an insulator, trapping your body heat and creating a microclimate that gets hotter as the night goes on. This is why you wake up sweating. The programmable solution is active thermal regulation. We now have mattress covers and smart beds that circulate water or air to strip heat away from the body. These systems can regulate the bed surface through the night and even develop feedback loops with wearable technologies.

Imagine a bed that knows you are in deep sleep and lowers the temperature to keep you there, then warms up slightly as your alarm time approaches to help you wake. We have some early peer reviewed studies that are now reporting modest but meaningful improvements in heart rate variability and deep sleep when the bed actively adjusts temperature. This is particularly vital for women going through menopause, where hot flashes can wreck sleep architecture. There is a vacuum here to be filled, and big bedding brands are moving quickly into this space. They know that a bed that stops you from sweating your sheets off at 2am is a bed you will pay a premium for.

The third element is sound. The sonic environment of the modern city is a disaster for sleep. Road noise, sirens, and the low frequency hum of urban life are constant intruders. Even if they do not fully wake you up, they can pull you out of deep sleep into lighter stages, fragmenting your recovery. The programmable room fights back with acoustic masking.

This is different from noise cancellation, which tries to erase sound. Masking adds a steady, broadband sound, often called pink or brown noise, that raises the acoustic floor of the room. This reduces the dynamic range between the background silence and the sudden spike of a slamming door or a passing motorbike. By smoothing out the peaks, the brain is less likely to trigger an arousal response. We are seeing the integration of smart soundscapes into bedroom hubs that can listen to the ambient noise level and adjust the masking volume in real time.

There is even research into closed loop auditory stimulation. This involves playing tiny, precise bursts of sound that are timed to the rising phase of the brain's slow waves during deep sleep. In the lab, this has been shown to boost slow wave activity and improve memory consolidation. It is like pushing a swing at the exact right moment to make it go higher. While the consumer tech for this is still maturing, the potential is clear. Sound becomes a tool to deepen sleep, not just something to block out.

Finally, there is the air itself. We often ignore air quality until it is visibly smoky, but invisible factors like carbon dioxide (CO_2) levels matter. In a small, sealed bedroom with the door and windows shut, CO_2 levels can rise significantly overnight just from your own breathing. High CO_2 is linked to stuffiness, poorer sleep quality, and that groggy feeling in the morning.

The programmable environment monitors this. Smart air purifiers and monitors can track particulate matter and CO_2. In a fully integrated smart home, a high CO_2 reading could trigger the HVAC system to cycle fresh air or even crack a motorised window. It ensures that the biosphere of the bedroom remains supportive of human life for the full eight hours.

The shift to the programmable environment is not just about gadgets. It is about recognising that the environment dictates behaviour and biology. We spend a third of our lives in this one room. It is the most important room in our lives for our health. Yet for decades, we have treated it with less technological sophistication than our kitchens or our cars.

We regulate the temperature of our fridges more precisely than we regulate the temperature of our sleeping children. That is changing. The bedroom is becoming a machine for rest. It is becoming a space where the walls, the lights, the bed, and the air all work in concert to support the singular biological goal of recovery.

This does not mean living in a spaceship. The best technology in this space will be invisible. It will be calm technology that recedes into the background. You will not be fiddling with apps or adjusting dials every night. You will simply walk into a room that feels right. The lights will be warm and dim. The air will be fresh. The bed will be cool. And when you lie down, the room will take care of the rest. The programmable environment is the stage, and you are the sleeper. The performance is about to begin.

The New Rules of Rest

We are living through the end of the era of intuitive sleep and ambient AI. For generations, the assessment of rest was a private, subjective affair. You woke up, stretched, and asked yourself a simple question: *How do I feel?* If you felt energised, you had slept well. If you felt groggy, you had slept poorly. It was a qualitative judgment, deeply personal and immune to external validation. No one could tell you that you were wrong about your own fatigue.

That simplicity has been replaced by a new regime of quantification. We have entered the age of the score. Today, for millions of people, the first act of the morning is not to check in with their bodies, but to check in with their data. We reach for the phone before we even leave the sheets. We look for a number, a Sleep Score of 85, a Readiness Rating of 42, a Recharge Percentage of 90. And in that split second of digital feedback, a strange and potent psychological shift occurs. The external metric overrides the internal sensation.

If the device says you slept poorly, but you actually feel fine, a seed of doubt is planted. You might suddenly start to feel heavier, slower. This is the nocebo effect of sleep tracking, the suggestion of a problem creating the symptoms of the problem. Conversely, if you feel terrible, perhaps you tossed and turned, or the room was too hot, but the device awards you a crown for excellent recovery because your heart rate variability remained high, you might push yourself harder than you should, ignoring your body's genuine distress signals. We are learning to trust the algorithm more than we trust our own nervous systems.

Sleep is a performance that refuses to be performed. It requires a surrender of control, a letting go of the conscious self. But the mindset of the tracker is all about control. It is about capturing, analysing, dissecting, and optimising. There is a fundamental tension between the manager mode of the day, which uses data to drive efficiency, and the sleeper mode of the night, which requires the absence of management. When we bring the manager into the bedroom, we often chase the sleeper away.

This does not mean we should discard the technology. It means we need to rewrite the rules of engagement. We need to develop a new data literacy for our own bodies. We must learn to treat these devices as compasses, not GPS systems. A compass is useful. It tells you if you are heading generally north or south. It helps you see trends over time, that alcohol ruins your recovery, or that a cool room improves it. But a GPS tells you exactly where you are to the inch, and consumer sleep trackers are simply not that precise yet. They are making estimates based on movement and blood flow, not reading your mind. If we treat their estimates as absolute truths, we set ourselves up for unnecessary anxiety and more sleep problems. Isn't it ironic?

Beyond the psychology of the individual, the new rules of rest are also being written by regulators. For the first decade of the wearable revolution, the industry operated in a comfortable grey zone known as wellness. Manufacturers promised to help you understand your rest or improve your habits, carefully avoiding any claim that they could diagnose or treat a medical condition. This linguistic dance kept them safe from the scrutiny of bodies like the Food and Drug Administration or the Therapeutic Goods Administration.

That era is closing. The grey zone is evaporating. We are witnessing the maturation of the market, driven by the realisation that sleep data is not just lifestyle trivia. It is health data. And if it is health data, it needs to be protected and regulated like a medical record.

The shift is visible in the actions of tech giants. They are no longer content with wellness labels. They want clinical validation. We are seeing a rush of regulatory clearances for features on consumer watches, from atrial fibrillation detection to sleep apnoea risk assessment. This is a massive pivot. When a consumer electronics company submits its algorithms to a federal health regulator, it signals the end of the toy phase. It means they are confident enough in the data to stake their legal liability on it.

This transition changes the stakes. For the consumer, it means the numbers on your wrist are starting to carry the weight of medical evidence. For the industry, it means the move fast and break things ethos of Silicon Valley is colliding with the first, do no harm ethos of medicine. You cannot beta test a pacemaker for the tongue.

We are already seeing devices that cross the line from passive tracking to active intervention. The FDA has cleared systems like NightWare, which runs on a smartwatch to treat PTSD related nightmares. It learns the wearer's physiology and delivers a gentle vibration to interrupt a nightmare without waking the user. This is a prescription therapy delivered via a consumer gadget. It closes the loop between sensing and treating.

But with great power comes great privacy risk. As our bedrooms become data factories, the question of ownership becomes critical. We have seen warning signs, like fitness apps inadvertently revealing military base locations through aggregated user data. Regulators are waking up to this. In the US, the Federal Trade Commission is cracking down on data brokers. In Europe, the AI Act prohibits the use of emotion AI in workplaces, preventing companies from using sleep data to gauge staff mood or engagement.

Governance is the boring secret that makes the sleep revolution sustainable. It provides the social licence for these technologies to exist in our intimate spaces. We need to know that the camera monitoring our breathing is not recording our conversations. We need to know that our insomnia data will not be sold to our life insurer.

We are moving toward a world where the bedroom is a regulated space. Not by a policeman in the corner, but by consumer protections that define what safe light, accurate sensing, and ethical data use look like. This is the end of the Wild West: the sleep economy is growing up.

Ultimately, the new rules of rest are about balance. We are the most measured humans in history, but we must not let the measurement obscure the magic. The best sensor you will ever own is your own brain. The best metric is how you feel at 11am. Technology is a powerful co-pilot, capable of spotting danger and optimising our environment. But it should never become the captain. The future of sleep is not about achieving a perfect score every night. It is about using the tools of the future to reclaim the ancient, rhythmic peace of the past, so we can finally do the one thing technology cannot do for us. Close our eyes and drift away.

2

Bodies Online at Bedtime

ATTRIBUTED TO GALILEO

The Internet of Bodies (IoB)

For centuries, sleep remained firmly in the category of things that were difficult to measure. It was a black box. You went into it, you experienced a period of lost time, and you emerged either refreshed or exhausted. The only data you had was your own subjective feeling upon waking. Doctors could only guess at what happened in the dark based on your descriptions of dreams or the bags under your eyes. To get real data, you had to go to a hospital, be wired up like a science fiction experiment, and try to sleep while strangers watched a bank of monitors. That era of mystery is over. We have taken Galileo's advice to heart and applied it to the most intimate third of our lives. We have entered the age of the Internet of Bodies: The IoB.

This concept takes the familiar idea of the Internet of Things and applies it to human biology. We are used to the Internet of Things. We accept that our fridge might be connected to the WiFi, that our doorbell has a camera we can check from work, and that our thermostat knows the local weather report. The Internet of Bodies is the next logical, if slightly unsettled, step. It is the moment when the network extends past the device and into the person. When you put on a smart ring, or strap a sensor to your chest, or lie down on a mattress that tracks your heart rate, you are turning your physical body into a node in a digital network. You are bringing your biology online.

It is not quite at the stage yet to read your mind (yet), but there are some technologies coming out so fast into the investor world that the landscape changes monthly. Smart wearables do not yet diagnose diseases, but they are much better than they used to be at gathering data and sharing it with medical providers. The Internet of Bodies at bedtime allows for the creation of a digital twin. This is a virtual model of your sleep physiology constructed from the streams of data your body produces. By connecting all these data points, the human body fully joins the network of the night. It allows for a level of insight that was previously impossible. We can see how a glass of wine at dinner affects our heart rate variability at 3am. We can see how a stressful day at work changes the temperature regulation of our skin during deep sleep. We can see the correlations between our lifestyle choices and our biological recovery.

This is a profound shift in self-knowledge. For most of history, we have been strangers to our own sleep. We knew we were tired, but we did not know why. We knew we dreamt, but we did not know when. Now, the Internet of Bodies shines a light into that dark cave. It gives us a map of the territory. It allows us to see the architecture of our rest.

However, this new visibility comes with new questions. If our bodies are online, who has access to the data? If our bedrooms are laboratories, who is running the experiment? The Internet of Bodies is not just a technological marvel; it is a social and ethical challenge. It blurs the line between the private self and the public network. It invites the algorithms of Silicon Valley into the most intimate moments of our lives.

The promise of the Internet of Bodies is that it will help us sleep better. It promises to use data to optimise our environment, to spot health problems before they become acute, and to guide us toward more restorative rest. But the risk is that it turns sleep into yet another performance metric, another thing to be managed, tracked, and optimised. It risks making us observers of our own sleep rather than participants in it.

As we build this network of sensors and signals, we must be careful to ensure that it serves us, and not the other way around. The goal should be to use the Internet of Bodies to support the biological body, to remove friction, and to create the conditions for deep, natural sleep. The technology should be the scaffolding, not the building itself. Ultimately, the measure of success for the Internet of Bodies will be whether it allows us to eventually forget about the data and just go to sleep. We are building a complex digital infrastructure so that, hopefully, we can return to a simple biological truth. We are wiring ourselves up so that we can finally switch off.

The Physics of Sensing

If you stripped away the sleek marketing, the brushed titanium finishes, and the monthly subscription apps, the technology currently tracking your sleep would look surprisingly humble. We often imagine that our devices are performing some kind of dark magic, peering into our souls to determine if we are rested. In reality, they are performing physics. They are measuring simple physical phenomena, i.e. light, motion, electrical resistance, and pressure, and using mathematics to guess what those signals mean for your biology.

To understand the Internet of Bodies, we have to look at the sensors themselves. How does a plastic disc on your wrist know that you are dreaming? The answer usually starts with a green light.

Most consumer wearables, from the ubiquitous smartwatches to the newer smart rings, rely on a technology called photoplethysmography, or PPG. While the name is a mouthful, the concept is elegant in its simplicity. Blood is red because it reflects red light and absorbs green light. Your heart beats, and with each beat, a fresh pulse of blood flows through your wrist or finger. When that pulse arrives, there is more blood in the capillaries, so more green light is absorbed. Between beats, there is less blood, and less absorption.

Your device is essentially shining a tiny flashlight into your skin hundreds of times a second and measuring the reflection. By tracking the rhythmic dimming and brightening of that reflected light, it can calculate your heart rate with impressive accuracy. On more advanced devices, different wavelengths of light, such as red and infrared, are used to estimate oxygen saturation (SpO2), peering deeper into the tissue to see how well your blood is carrying oxygen.

This optical physics provides a window into the autonomic nervous system. It allows the device to calculate Heart Rate Variability (HRV), which is the variation in time between each heartbeat. A metronomic heart often signals stress or engagement, while a heart with high variability indicates a system that is relaxed and ready to recover. This is one of the primary signals that algorithms use to determine if your body is truly resting or if it is still fighting the stress of the day.

However, light is not the only tool in the box. The second pillar of sleep sensing is motion, measured by an accelerometer. These are tiny electromechanical devices that detect proper acceleration as movement and gravity. In the early days of sleep tracking, this was the only metric. If you were moving, the device assumed you were awake. If you were still, it assumed you were asleep.

Today, accelerometers are far more sensitive. They can pick up the microscopic movements of your wrist as you shift positions, the tremors of a restless leg, or the stillness of deep paralysis during REM sleep. When combined with a microphone, they can also listen for the sonic signature of the night: snoring, coughing, or the silence of an apnoea event.

But what if you do not want to wear anything at all? This is where the physics shifts from optics to mechanics. Under-mattress sensors and smart mats use a technique called ballistocardiography. Every time your heart beats, it ejects blood into the aorta with significant force. Newton's third law of motion dictates that for every action, there is an equal and opposite reaction. This means that with every heartbeat, your entire body recoils slightly.

These micro-movements are invisible to the naked eye, but they are seismic events to a piezoelectric sensor placed under your mattress. These mats listen to the mechanical thump of your heart and the rhythmic rise and fall of your chest as you breathe. Because they are measuring mechanical force rather than optical reflection, they are often less confused by skin tone or tattoos, but they face their own challenges. If a pet jumps on the bed, or a partner rolls over, the sensor has to disentangle your heartbeat from the chaos of the environment.

Finally, we have the gold standard of electrical sensing: Electroencephalography (EEG). This is what happens in a sleep lab. Electrodes are glued to the scalp to measure the ionic current voltage fluctuations resulting from ionic current within the neurons of the brain. This is the only way to truly see sleep stages.

Consumer devices are trying to bridge this gap. We now have headbands that use dry electrodes to pick up brain rhythms without the messy conductive paste used in hospitals. These devices are getting closer to the ground truth of what the brain is doing, rather than just inferring it from the heart and lungs.

The challenge lies in synthesis. When you put all these streams together, e.g. the green light on the wrist, the motion of the accelerometer, the temperature reading from the finger, the algorithms attempt to draw a portrait of your sleep.

Right now, that portrait is more of a graphite sketch than a high-definition photograph. A smart watch does not read brain waves; it infers sleep stages from secondary signals. It guesses that you are in REM sleep because your body is paralysed (accelerometer) but your heart rate is elevated (PPG). It guesses you are in deep sleep because your heart rate has slowed and your variability has synchronised with your breathing.

This inference is clever, and for many people, it works most of the time. Independent studies show that modern wearables are actually quite good at the big picture: determining if you are asleep or awake, and calculating your total sleep time. Where they struggle is the granular detail. They often confuse quiet wakefulness, lying in bed reading or thinking, with light sleep. They can struggle to differentiate between REM and light sleep because the heart rate signals can look similar.

There are also physical limitations to the sensors themselves. Optical sensors can struggle with darker skin tones, leading to inaccuracies in heart rate and oxygen readings. They can be confused by tattoos, which block the light, or by cold hands, which constrict the capillaries and hide the pulse. Accelerometers can be tricked by a restless partner or puppy.

This is the reality of the physics of sensing. We are using external proxies to guess at internal states. We are shining lights, listening for thumps, and measuring wiggles, and then using advanced mathematics to turn that noisy data into a neat graph on your phone screen. It is a technological marvel, but it is not magic. It is an estimation.

Understanding this physics is the best defence against anxiety about sleep data. When you know that your deep sleep score is an algorithmic guess based on your pulse, rather than a direct readout of your brain, you can hold the data a little more lightly. You can look at the trends rather than obsess over the nightly score. You can appreciate the sketch for what it is; a useful guide, not a perfect portrait.

As we move forward, these sensors will evolve. We are seeing the rise of radar that can sense breathing without touching you, and earbuds that measure brainwaves from the ear canal. The resolution and granularity of the data is improving every year. But for now, it is enough to know that the device on your wrist is just a very clever observer, using the basic laws of physics to try and understand the complex mystery of your sleep.

Invisible and Internal

For many people, the biggest barrier to tracking sleep is the tracker itself. There is an inherent friction in strapping a computer to your wrist before you go to bed. It requires charging. It can feel bulky or hot against the skin. It lights up in the middle of the night. And for some, the very act of putting it on signals a performance mindset that makes sleep harder to achieve. The industry has recognised this fatigue, and the response has been a shift towards technology that disappears. We are moving from wearables to nearables, and even further, to implantables.

This is the frontier of invisible sensing. One of the most futuristic examples of this is bedside radar. It sounds like something from an aviation manual, but low-power radar chips are now sitting on nightstands in suburban bedrooms. Technologies like Google's Soli radar use electromagnetic waves to detect movement on a sub-millimetre scale. These waves travel from the device, bounce off the sleeper, and return to the sensor. By analysing the shift in the returning waves, the device can detect the rhythmic rise and fall of a chest as it breathes.

It can do this through a duvet. It can do it in pitch darkness. It does not need a camera, which preserves a degree of privacy that many users find essential in a bedroom setting. Independent studies have shown that these contactless systems can estimate heart rate and respiratory rate with surprising accuracy, and they are excellent at detecting the large movements that signal restlessness or wakefulness. For the person who cannot tolerate a watch, or for the partner who refuses to participate in the quantified self-experiment, radar offers a passive, silent observer.

However, radar has its blind spots. It tracks the closest moving object. If a large dog jumps on the bed, or if two sleepers cuddle too closely, the signal can become confused. It struggles to distinguish between two people in a shared bed without careful calibration. It is a distance sensor, and distance in a bed is a variable concept.

At the other end of the spectrum, technology is crossing the skin barrier entirely. For people with serious sleep disorders, the internet of bodies is becoming literal. We are seeing the rise of implantable sleep technologies that do not just measure sleep but actively engineer it.

The most prominent of these is hypoglossal nerve stimulation. This is a therapy for obstructive sleep apnoea, a condition where the tongue and soft tissues collapse during sleep, blocking the airway. For decades, the gold standard treatment has been Continuous Positive Airway Pressure (CPAP), a machine that blows air through a mask to keep the throat open. But many patients struggle with the mask. It is intrusive, loud, and uncomfortable.

Hypoglossal nerve stimulation offers a bionic alternative. A surgeon implants a small device, similar to a pacemaker, in the chest. A lead wire is tunnelled up the neck to the hypoglossal nerve, which controls the movement of the tongue. When the patient goes to sleep, they turn the device on with a small remote. The device monitors breathing, and just before the patient inhales, it delivers a mild electrical pulse to the nerve. This pulse causes the tongue to stiffen and move slightly forward, opening the airway mechanically from the inside.

This is a profound integration of man and machine. The technology is essentially hijacking the body's own nervous system to maintain breathing. It transforms a mechanical problem of collapsing tissue into a software problem that can be solved with electricity. Long-term data shows that these devices are safe and effective, providing a lifeline for people who cannot tolerate external masks.

We are also seeing similar technology for central sleep apnoea, a condition where the brain fails to send the signal to breathe. Devices like the remedē system stimulate the phrenic nerve to contract the diaphragm, breathing for the patient when their own brain forgets to do so. This is the Internet of Bodies operating at the level of the brainstem.

The move towards invisible and implantable tech represents a maturing of the sleep economy. It acknowledges that for technology to be truly useful, it must be frictionless. It must work when we are unconscious, uncooperative, and unencumbered. Whether it is a radar dish watching from the side or a pacemaker humming in the chest, the future of sleep tracking is not about what we wear. It is about where we are. We are building a nest that knows us, and for the first time, we are inviting the machine inside.

The Edges of Accuracy

When you open your sleep app in the morning, you are presented with a masterpiece of certainty. The interface is likely crisp and authoritative, displaying your sleep stages in bright, colour-coded blocks. It tells you that you had exactly forty-two minutes of deep sleep, that your REM cycle started at 3:14am, and that your overall 'Readiness Score' is an 85. It looks like a medical diagnosis. It feels like absolute truth.

But if you were to peel back the glossy interface and look at the raw data, you would see something far messier. You would see a chaotic stream of signal and noise, full of gaps, guesses, and approximations. This is the dirty secret of the sleep economy: the devices are confident, but they are not always right. Understanding where these devices fail is just as important as understanding how they work. We need to know where the edges of accuracy lie so that we do not fall off them.

The first and most serious limitation is one of physics and biology intersecting with design bias. As we discussed, most wearables use green light photoplethysmography (PPG) to read heart rate. The sensor shines light into the skin and measures what bounces back. However, the physics of light absorption changes depending on the colour of the canvas. Melanin, the pigment that gives skin its colour, absorbs light. Higher levels of melanin can reduce the amount of light that returns to the sensor, creating a weaker signal-to-noise ratio.

For years, clinical pulse oximetry faced a reckoning over this exact issue, where devices often overestimated oxygen levels in patients with darker skin, potentially masking hypoxemia. Consumer wearables have inherited this challenge. While algorithms have improved, studies continue to show that optical heart rate sensors can be less accurate on darker skin tones, particularly during moments of high activity or rapid heart rate change. This means that the universal technology of the sleep revolution is not actually working equally for everyone. A device that works perfectly for a pale-skinned engineer in Silicon Valley might struggle to read the resting heart rate of a dark-skinned shift worker in Brisbane. If the foundational signal is shaky, every metric built on top of it, from sleep stages to recovery scores, becomes suspect.

Then there is the tattoo problem. Ink sits in the dermis, the same layer of skin where the blood vessels reside. Dark ink, particularly solid black bands often found on wrists, can block the green light entirely, effectively blinding the sensor. Users with wrist tattoos often find their expensive smartwatches failing to record any heart rate data at all, or producing wild inaccuracies. It is a reminder that these devices were designed for a standardised, unblemished human body that exists in a lab, not necessarily the varied and decorated bodies that exist in the real world.

Beyond the skin, there is the problem of behaviour. Sleep trackers are fundamentally guessing games. They do not know you are asleep; they infer it from a lack of movement and a slowing heart. But sleep is not the only time we are still and calm. If you lie in bed for an hour reading a book, or watching a movie with a low heart rate, your device will almost certainly log that time as light sleep.

This inability to distinguish between quiet wakefulness and actual sleep is the Achilles' heel of consumer tracking. It creates a phenomenon where the device overestimates your sleep duration. You might wake up feeling groggy because you lay awake for two hours, but your app congratulates you on a solid eight-hour night. This gaslighting can be incredibly frustrating. It creates a dissonance between your lived experience and your digital record. You know you were awake; the machine says you were asleep. Who do you trust?

The algorithms also struggle with the chaotic reality of shared beds. A motion sensor on your wrist or a mat under your mattress is sensitive to vibration. It cannot tell the difference between your movement and the movement of a partner rolling over, or a large dog jumping up at 3am, or a toddler climbing in after a nightmare. The signal of your sleep is constantly polluted by the noise of your environment.

Under-mattress sensors are particularly vulnerable to this. While they are excellent at being invisible, they are measuring the mechanical physics of the entire bed surface. If your partner has restless legs, your sleep score might plummet, even if you slept like a log. The device attributes the vibration to you. Radar systems face a similar challenge, sometimes locking onto the wrong person if two sleepers are close together. The technology assumes a solitary sleeper in a sterile box, but human sleep is often communal and messy.

Perhaps the most subtle but pervasive inaccuracy lies in sleep staging. We all want to know how much deep sleep and REM we are getting. But identifying these stages accurately requires reading brain waves (using EEG) and eye movements (EOG). A watch on the wrist has access to neither. It is trying to reverse-engineer the brain's state by looking at the heart's shadow.

While there is a correlation (heart rate tends to be lowest and most regular in deep sleep, and variable in REM) it is not a perfect map. Independent validation studies comparing wearables to gold-standard polysomnography often show accuracy rates for sleep staging hovering around 60 to 70 per cent. That is better than a coin toss, but it is hardly a medical diagnostic. The device might tell you that you got zero deep sleep last night, causing you to panic about your brain health, when in reality it simply missed the subtle heart rate signals that mark that stage.

This leads us to the final and most dangerous edge of accuracy: the psychological impact of the data itself. We have discussed orthosomnia, the anxiety caused by tracking, but it is worth revisiting here as a limitation of the technology. The device is not a neutral observer. By presenting data, it changes the outcome.

When a device presents a red recovery score or a low readiness rating, it is delivering a nocebo: a negative suggestion. If you wake up feeling okay, but your phone tells you that your recovery is terrible, you may subconsciously adopt that fatigue. You may skip the gym, be less patient with your kids, or perform worse at work, all because a piece of plastic on your wrist made a calculation based on a slightly elevated heart rate. The inaccuracy of the device becomes a self-fulfilling prophecy.

This is where the human in the loop becomes essential. We must learn to treat these devices as advisors, not judges. We need to look at the data through the lens of context. *My heart rate was high? well, I had three glasses of wine. My deep sleep was low? Well, the cat slept on my legs. My readiness is zero? Well, I feel great, so I'm going for a run anyway.*

The technology is amazing, but it is brittle. It breaks when confronted with tattoos, dark skin, reading in bed, pets, and the complex variability of human physiology. It provides a sketch, not a photograph. As long as we treat it as a sketch, a rough outline of our night, it can be incredibly useful. But if we mistake it for a high-definition truth, we risk letting the edges of the technology cut into the quality of our rest. The map is not the territory, and the sleep score is not the sleep.

The Digital Twin and Interoperability

We are approaching the final frontier of the Internet of Bodies, and it is not a physical device you wear or a sensor you sleep on. It is a mathematical model. It is the moment when the streams of data from your wrist, your mattress, your thermostat, and your medical history converge to create a virtual copy of your physiology. This is the era of the Digital Twin.

In engineering, a digital twin is a standard concept. Before a manufacturer builds a jet engine, they build a perfect digital replica of it in a computer. They run millions of simulations on the twin, i.e. subjecting it to extreme heat, stress, and turbulence, to predict how the real engine will perform before it even exists in the physical world. It allows them to crash the plane in the simulator so they do not have to crash it in the real world.

Now, researchers and tech companies are applying this same logic to human sleep. The goal is to build a circadian digital twin of you. This twin is not just a log of how you slept last night; it is a dynamic, predictive model of how your specific body responds to the world. It learns your unique phase response curve, i.e. how sensitive you are to light at 10pm versus

7am. It learns how fast you metabolise caffeine. It learns the thermal signature of your deep sleep.

Once the model is robust, it moves from observation to simulation. This is the pilot simulator for your sleep. Imagine you have a flight from Perth to London coming up next week. Instead of guessing when to sleep or drink coffee, you feed the flight details into your digital twin. The system runs thousands of scenarios, testing different light exposure schedules and nap times. It finds the optimal path that results in the least amount of jet lag for your specific biology, and then pushes that plan to your phone. It allows you to make the mistakes in silico, so you do not have to make them in real life.

This capability extends to therapy as well. For a shift worker, the digital twin could simulate the coming roster. It could predict that a specific rotation will cause a dangerous drop in alertness at 3am on Tuesday, and proactively suggest a preventative nap or a specific light exposure window to shift the body clock in advance. It turns sleep medicine from a reactive discipline, effectively treating the exhaustion after it happens, into a predictive one.

However, for a digital twin to exist, the data has to be able to flow. This brings us to the boring secret that makes the entire sleep economy possible: interoperability.

For years, the sleep tech landscape was a series of walled gardens. Your smart ring data lived in one app, your smart mattress data lived in another, and your medical records lived in a filing cabinet at your doctor's office. None of these systems spoke the same language. Your thermostat had no idea you were in deep sleep, so it kept the room too hot. Your doctor had no idea you were using a smart ring, so they relied on your hazy memory of how you slept.

This fragmentation is ending. We are seeing a push towards open standards and shared languages for health data. Technologies like Health Connect on Android and the Health framework on Apple devices act as bridges, allowing different apps to swap data securely. Even more importantly, we are seeing the adoption of clinical standards like Fast Healthcare Interoperability Resources (FHIR), which allow consumer data to flow into professional medical systems.

This interoperability is the magic key. It means that your smart ring can share your total sleep time and respiratory rate directly with a research study or a telehealth service. It means your lighting system can read your circadian phase from your wearable and adjust the colour temperature of the bulbs automatically. When the systems talk to each other, the programmable environment we discussed earlier finally becomes real. The bed tells the lights to dim; the watch tells the thermostat to cool; the phone tells the coffee machine to wait. The user does not have to act as the system administrator for their own bedroom.

This connection to the medical world is critical. We are moving to a model where the bedroom is an extension of the clinic. *Hospital at Home* programs are already using remote monitoring to care for patients in their own beds. During the pandemic, this was a necessity; now, it is a strategy. Pulse oximeters and sleep mats allow clinicians to monitor recovery from the safety of a dashboard.

But this connected future brings us back to the question of control. If your digital twin lives in the cloud, who owns it? If your sleep data flows seamlessly to your insurance company, can they use it to raise your premiums because you stay up too late?

The Internet of Bodies is not just about gadgets; it is about rights. As we build these digital twins, we need digital rights to match. We need the right to delete our data. We need the right to know who is seeing it. We need the right to portability, to take our digital twin from one platform to another, just as we can take our phone number to a new carrier.

Regulators are beginning to sharpen their tools. We are seeing moves to treat sleep data as sensitive health information, regardless of whether it was collected by a medical device or a consumer toy. The social licence for these technologies depends on trust. If people feel that their digital twin is being used to spy on them rather than support them, they will simply take the watch off.

Ultimately, the goal of the Internet of Bodies, the physics of sensing, and the digital twin is to give you something rare in medicine: control in your own hands. It offers the promise that you can understand the black box of your own sleep.

It suggests that with enough data, and enough processing power, we can finally decode the night.

But we must remember that the map is not the territory. A digital twin is a model, not a human. It cannot capture the feeling of a cold pillow on a hot night, or the comfort of a heavy blanket, or the strange logic of a dream. It is a tool, a powerful co-pilot, but it is not the pilot.

As we close this chapter on the connected body, the invitation is to use these tools wisely. Use the sensors to spot apnoea. Use the digital twin to plan your travel. Use the interoperability to automate your lights. But do not let the data obscure the simple, biological truth. You are not a node in a network. You are a human being who needs to rest. The technology is there to serve the sleep, not the other way around. The best outcome of the Internet of Bodies is that it works so well, and so quietly, that you eventually feel safe enough to disconnect, close your eyes, and go offline.

3

AI as Your Sleep Co-Pilot

From Tracking to Coaching

There is a deafening amount of noise when it comes to sleep advice. If you have ever mentioned at a dinner party or a school gate that you are feeling tired, you will know exactly what happens next. Everyone has an opinion. You will be told to try magnesium, or to tape your mouth shut, or to buy a weighted blanket, or to drink tart cherry juice. You will be told to wake up at 5am to join the hustle culture, or to sleep in to honour your body. The internet is even louder, filled with influencers and experts offering masterclasses on the perfect morning routine, and typically they are young men with no children in their care.

Most of this advice is well meaning, and some of it is even scientifically sound. But almost all of it suffers from a fatal flaw. It is generic. It is a one size fits all approach applied to a biological function that is as individual as a fingerprint. Telling everyone to go to bed at 10pm is like telling everyone to wear a size medium shoe. It will work for some, it will be uncomfortable for others, and for a few, it will be completely debilitating.

This is where the role of technology is shifting fundamentally. For the last ten years, sleep tech has been stuck in the era of tracking. We have become very good at recording what happened. We wake up, we look at a graph that tells us we tossed and turned at 2am, and we think, yes, I know, I was there. This is rear view mirror data. It confirms the past, but it does very little to change the future. Knowing you slept poorly is not the same as knowing how to sleep better.

Artificial Intelligence is now cracking this problem open. It is moving the industry from the era of tracking to the era of coaching. We are transitioning from passive observation to active guidance. If the wearable of the last decade was a scorecard, the wearable of the next decade is a co-pilot.

Think of the difference between a car dashboard and a satellite navigation system. The dashboard tells you how fast you are going and how much fuel you have left. That is useful information, but it does not help you get to your destination. The navigation system, however, knows where you want to go. It looks at the traffic ahead, it calculates the best route, and it gives you specific, timely instructions. *Turn left in 100 metres. Slow down, hazard ahead.*

This is the promise of AI in the bedroom. It is a system that watches the dials of your biology so you do not have to. It runs simulations, makes predictions, and then nudges your behaviour and your environment so that your brain can land the plane safely in the destination of a good night's sleep.

The power of this co-pilot lies in its ability to handle complexity. Human sleep is influenced by dozens of variables. It is shaped by the light you saw this morning, the coffee you drank at lunch, the temperature of your room, the stress of your email inbox, and the timing of your dinner. It is also shaped by your unique genetic chronotype and your age. No human being can calculate the interaction of all these variables in their head every single day. We are bad at spotting long term patterns in noisy data. We might think that cheese gives us nightmares because we remember the one time it happened, but we miss the fact that every time we exercise after 7pm, our deep sleep drops by ten per cent.

AI models thrive on this kind of mess. Give a model several weeks of your light exposure, wrist movements, heart rhythms, and bedtime patterns, and it can start to map out your personal path to sleep. These models do not read your dreams or your mind, but they are excellent at finding regularities that your eyes miss. They can turn those hidden patterns into simple steps you can try tonight.

For example, a generic health article might tell you that caffeine has a half-life of five hours and you should stop drinking it at noon. But your AI co-pilot, having analysed your specific data for a month (maybe from your smart toilet), might see that you are actually a fast metaboliser. It might tell you that you can safely have a coffee at 2pm without impacting your sleep onset latency. Or, conversely, it might notice that on days you have a second cup, your REM sleep fragments, and suggest a stricter cut off than the average person needs. This moves the advice from *people should do this* to *you should do this*. It personalises the protocol. It treats you as an experiment of one.

The co-pilot metaphor extends to how the system interacts with you. A good co-pilot is not annoying. It does not nag you constantly. It speaks up only when it matters. In the past, health apps were guilty of spamming users with generic notifications. *Time to wind down! Did you sleep well? Drink water!* We learned to ignore them because they were not relevant to our immediate context.

The next generation of AI tools is context aware. They use the sensors we discussed in the previous chapters to know what is happening right now. If your digital co-pilot sees that you have had a particularly stressful day, evidenced by high heart rate variability and a lack of movement, it might adjust your evening plan. Instead of pushing you to do a heavy workout, it might suggest a restorative walk and an earlier bedtime. If it knows you have a flight to London tomorrow, it might start shifting your light exposure schedule three days in advance to mitigate the coming jet lag.

This is the shift from a static rulebook to a dynamic strategy. Sleep is not a steady state. It fluctuates with the seasons, with our hormones, with our work schedules, and with our age. A rigid routine often breaks when life gets messy. An AI co-pilot adapts. It recalculates the route when you miss a turn. If you stay up late for a birthday party, it does not just shame you for missing your bedtime. It looks at the data and suggests the best way to recover the next day. Maybe it tells you to sleep in for an extra forty five minutes, or maybe it tells you to get up at your usual time but take a twenty minute nap at 1pm.

We are seeing this capability emerge in high performance environments first. Pilots on ultra long haul flights use fatigue risk management systems that predict their alertness levels hours in advance. These systems tell them exactly when to take a controlled rest in the bunk so that they will be peak alert for landing. Now, that same logic is coming to the consumer. You do not have to be flying a Boeing 747 to benefit from fatigue management. You just have to be a parent, a shift worker, or an executive trying to make good decisions.

The mechanism behind this is not magic. It is pattern recognition at scale. The AI is constantly comparing your current state to your historical baseline. It is looking for deviations. It notices that your resting heart rate is creeping up, which might signal an incoming illness or a need for recovery. It notices that your room temperature is two degrees higher than your historical average for deep sleep, and flags it.

This allows for a proactive approach to sleep health. Instead of waiting until you are exhausted and burnt out to seek help, the co-pilot can flag the trend early. It can show you that your sleep debt is accumulating before you feel the full weight of it. It can act as an early warning system for your own biology.

Ultimately, the goal of the AI co-pilot is to reduce the cognitive load of sleep. We spend so much energy worrying about whether we are doing the right things. We do mental math about coffee times and gym sessions. We stress about whether we will be tired tomorrow. The co-pilot offloads this anxiety. It takes responsibility for the logistics of the night. It watches the clock and the sensors so you do not have to. It allows you to trust that there is a plan, and that the plan is tailored specifically to you.

As we move through this chapter, we will look at exactly how these models work, where they succeed, and where they can hallucinate or fail. But the headline is clear. The era of the dumb tracker is over. The era of the intelligent agent has arrived. And for anyone who has ever stared at a ceiling wondering why they cannot sleep, having a co-pilot in the room might just be the change that finally makes a difference.

Algorithmic Sleep Staging

When you wake up and look at your phone, you are usually presented with a neat, colour coded bar chart known as a hypnogram. It slices your night into tidy blocks of light sleep, deep sleep, REM sleep, and wakefulness. It looks authoritative, precise, and scientific. It implies that the device on your wrist spent the night watching your brain with the accuracy of a neuroscientist.

The reality is that your device was doing no such thing. It was guessing. To be more charitable, it was inferring. This process is called algorithmic sleep staging, and it represents one of the most complex challenges in the entire sleep economy. It is the attempt to translate the noisy, physical movements of the wrist and the rhythmic pulsing of blood in the capillaries into a map of the electrical storms happening inside your skull.

To understand how this works, and why it sometimes fails, we have to look at how sleep staging is supposed to be done. In a clinical sleep lab, a technician uses a method that has barely changed in decades. They glue electrodes to your scalp, face, and chest to record your brain waves (EEG), eye movements (EOG), and muscle tone (EMG). These signals are fed into a computer, which displays them as squiggly lines on a screen.

The technician then goes through the entire night's recording, slicing it into thirty second chunks called epochs. For each epoch, they look at the squiggles and apply a strict set of rules. If they see slow, high amplitude waves, they mark it as deep sleep. If they see rapid, low voltage waves and rapid eye movements, they mark it as REM. It is a manual, laborious process. It is the gold standard, but it is also subjective. Two human experts scoring the same night will disagree with each other from time to time.

Your smart watch cannot do this. It has no access to your brain waves or your eye movements. It is effectively blind to the primary signals of sleep. Instead, it relies on secondary proxies. It measures your heart rate, your heart rate variability, your movement, and sometimes your temperature or respiration rate.

This is where the artificial intelligence comes in. The algorithm in your watch has been trained on massive datasets. The manufacturers take thousands of people, put them in a sleep lab with full EEG wiring, and also strap the wearable device to their wrists. They then feed both streams of data (the brain waves and the wrist signals) into a machine learning model.

The model essentially plays a game of pattern matching. It asks itself questions like: *When the heart rate drops and the variability stabilises, and the accelerometer shows zero movement for ten minutes, what is the brain usually doing?* The answer, statistically, is usually deep sleep. *When the heart rate becomes erratic and climbs slightly, but the body is completely paralysed, what is the brain usually doing?* That is usually REM.

Over millions of epochs of training, the model learns the statistical probabilities. It learns that a certain pattern of pulse and stillness correlates with light sleep eighty per cent of the time. When you wear the device at home, it is applying these learned probabilities to your live data. It is not seeing your sleep; it is predicting it based on what it saw in the training data.

The problem is that human biology is messy. The correlation between heart rate and brain state is strong, but it is not perfect. There are moments of quiet wakefulness, perhaps lying in bed reading or meditating, where the heart rate slows and the body is still. To the algorithm, this looks exactly like the onset of sleep. This is why trackers often overestimate how much sleep you are getting; they struggle to tell the difference between rest and unconsciousness.

Similarly, the autonomic signatures of REM sleep and light sleep can overlap. Both can involve variable heart rates. Without the tell-tale sign of rapid eye movements which the watch cannot see, the algorithm has to make a best guess. This is why you might see your REM score fluctuate wildly from night to night, or why different devices on the same wrist can give you different sleep stages for the same night. They are using different mathematical models to interpret the same physical signals.

For a long time, these consumer algorithms were black boxes. The companies protected them as trade secrets, making it impossible for independent scientists to verify how they worked.

We just had to trust the pretty graph. But this is changing. The rise of open source science is pushing the field towards transparency.

Newer, academic grade models like UC Berkeley's Yet Another Spindle Algorithm (YASA) and USleep (from University of Copenhagen) have been developed by researchers to show what is possible. These models are trained on tens of thousands of nights of data from diverse populations. They use deep learning to classify sleep stages with a level of consistency that rivals human scorers. USleep, for example, showed strong performance across multiple clinical cohorts, even when the data channels were not ideal. YASA offers fast, accurate staging from EEG and common biosignals, and because the code is open, the scientific community can scrutinise it, test it, and improve it.

This shift towards transparency matters because it helps us understand the limits of the tool. Validation studies comparing modern wearables against the clinical gold standard show that the best devices are now getting quite good at the basics. They can distinguish sleep from wake with high accuracy (sensitivity), and they are decent at spotting deep sleep. But they often struggle with the transitions. The minute by minute architecture of the night, i.e. exactly when you slipped from Stage 2 to REM, is often a rough approximation.

It is important to understand that these errors are not hallucinations in the AI sense; they are inference errors. The model is making a statistical bet that turns out to be wrong. It is treating your night as a probability distribution.

So, how should you use this imperfect tool? You should treat the hypnogram as a sketch, not a photograph. It captures the shape of your night, but not every detail. If the device says you got three hours of deep sleep, you can be confident you had a restorative night. If it says you got three minutes, you can be confident something disrupted you. But if it says you entered REM at 3:14am and exited at 3:22am, you should take that precision with a grain of salt.

The value of algorithmic staging is not in the minute by minute accuracy of a single night. It is in the trend. If you usually get an hour of deep sleep, and then you start drinking alcohol before bed and that number drops to thirty minutes and stays there for a week, that is a real signal. The algorithm might be imperfect, but it is consistently imperfect. It detects the change in your baseline.

We are moving towards a future where these algorithms will get smarter. They will start to incorporate more data points, perhaps from bedside radar or temperature sensors, to triangulate the sleep stage with higher fidelity. But until we have cheap, comfortable EEG sensors that we can wear on our foreheads every night, we are relying on a proxy.

Personalised Circadian Modelling

If you have ever tried to force yourself to sleep before a big flight, or stared at the ceiling at 4am after crossing time zones, you have met your circadian rhythm. It is the silent, internal conductor that orchestrates every biological system in your body. It decides when you release hormones, when your body temperature drops, when your digestion slows down, and critically, when you are capable of falling asleep.

For most of the history of sleep science, measuring this internal clock was a difficult and messy process. To know exactly where your body clock was set, a clinician would have to perform a test called the Dim Light Melatonin Onset, or DLMO. This involves sitting in a dimly lit lab for hours, chewing on cotton swabs or giving blood samples every thirty to sixty minutes to detect the precise moment your pineal gland starts secreting melatonin. It is accurate, but it is expensive, uncomfortable, and completely impractical for daily life.

Because we could not measure the clock easily, we ignored it. We gave generic advice based on social time, not biological time. We told people to go to bed at a reasonable hour, assuming that 10pm means the same thing to a night owl teenager as it does to an early bird grandmother. We treated time as a rigid, external scaffolding that the body had to climb, rather than an internal fluid process.

Artificial Intelligence is changing this. We are moving from the era of guessing your timing to the era of modelling it. This is the domain of Personalised Circadian Modelling. It is the mathematical attempt to find the hidden variable of your circadian phase without needing a saliva sample.

The breakthrough comes from realising that your body clock leaves fingerprints all over your physiology. It influences your resting heart rate, which tends to dip to its lowest point during the biological night. It drives the daily fluctuation of your skin temperature. It dictates your patterns of movement and stillness. By feeding these streams of data from a wearable device into a sophisticated machine learning model, researchers have found that they can estimate your circadian phase with surprising accuracy.

This effectively turns your smart watch into a proxy for a melatonin test. The AI looks at the history of your light exposure, your activity, and your heart rhythm over the last few weeks, and it calculates where your internal midnight actually sits. It might tell you that while the clock on the wall says 11pm, your body thinks it is only 9pm. This explains why you are wide awake and frustrated. You are not an insomniac; you are simply trying to sleep in your biological evening.

Once the AI knows your phase, it can start to build something even more powerful: a digital twin of you and you alone. In engineering, a digital twin is a virtual replica of a physical system, used to run simulations. NASA uses them for spacecraft; Formula One teams use them for cars. Now, sleep scientists are building them for people. A circadian digital twin is a mathematical model of your specific body clock. It learns how sensitive you are to light. It learns how fast your clock shifts in response to travel. It creates a sandbox where the AI can test different strategies before you try them in real life.

Imagine you are a shift worker about to rotate from a day schedule to a night schedule. This is usually a brutal transition that results in profound fatigue and safety risks. A standard roster might just tell you to show up at 7pm. But your AI co-pilot, running your digital twin, would approach it differently. It would simulate the week ahead. It would ask: *What happens if we push the sleep window two hours later on Tuesday? What happens if we blast bright light for twenty minutes on Thursday morning?*

It runs these *what if* scenarios thousands of times in seconds, looking for the path that results in the highest alertness during the shift and the best recovery after it. It then presents you with a personalised plan. It might say: *On Wednesday, wear dark glasses on your drive home. On Thursday, get twenty minutes of sunlight as soon as you wake up. Do not drink coffee after 4am.*

This is the digital siblings approach. The model generates thousands of potential versions of your week, simulating the outcomes for each one, and then picks the sibling that had the best sleep. It allows you to optimise your schedule mathematically. This technology is particularly transformative for jet lag. Jet lag is essentially a math problem. It is a mismatch between your internal phase and the external solar day. The fastest way to solve the problem is with light, but the timing of that light is critical. Light at the wrong time can actually push your clock in the wrong direction, making the jet lag worse.

An AI co-pilot removes the guesswork. Several research groups have used control theory (the same mathematics used to guide missiles and robots) to compute time optimal light schedules. These are precise plans that shift the body clock to a new time zone in the mathematically shortest possible time. Instead of vaguely trying to stay awake until local bedtime, the app might tell you to seek bright light at 10am and avoid it strictly at 4pm. It turns the nebulous advice of 'get some sun' into a prescription as precise as a drug dosage.

We are also seeing this logic applied to the bedroom environment itself. Once the system knows your circadian phase, it can automate the room to support it. If your digital twin calculates that your melatonin onset is delayed, it might signal your smart lights to dim earlier and shift to a warmer spectrum to help pull your clock forward. It creates a feedback loop between your biology and your building.

This level of personalisation matters because the average human does not exist. A lighting schedule that helps an early bird might wreck the sleep of a night owl. A nap at 2pm might be restorative for one person and destroy the night's sleep for another. By modelling the individual, AI moves us away from the tyranny of the average.

There are limitations, of course. These models depend on the quality of the data. If you take your watch off for three days, or if the heart rate sensor is inaccurate, the digital twin will drift away from reality. The model is only as good as the signal. There is also the risk of over-optimisation, where we become slaves to a schedule that is mathematically perfect but socially impossible. We cannot always wear dark glasses at a wedding just because an algorithm told us to (although it might make you mysterious and interesting as a guest).

However, the direction of travel is clear. We are moving towards a world where we no longer have to guess what time it is inside our own bodies. The AI co-pilot provides a dashboard for our internal time. It reveals the hidden rhythm that governs our energy, our mood, and our sleep. And by making that rhythm visible, it gives us the power to work with it, rather than constantly fighting against it.

For the shift worker, the frequent flyer, and the parent of a newborn, this is not just a gadget. It is a tool for survival. It validates the reality that we are biological machines running on ancient hardware in a modern world. It acknowledges that timing is everything. And for the first time, it gives us a watch that actually knows what time it is.

The Risk of Hallucination

If you ask a modern artificial intelligence chatbot how to fix your insomnia, it will almost certainly give you an answer. It will likely be a very good answer, written in perfect, empathetic prose. It might suggest a protocol of sleep restriction, followed by a stimulus control strategy, perhaps peppered with advice about magnesium or blue light. It will sound authoritative, confident, and uncannily human. It will sound exactly like a doctor.

But it is not a doctor. It is a probabilistic engine that predicts the next likely word in a sentence. And this distinction brings us to the most dangerous frontier of the AI sleep revolution: the risk of hallucination.

In the context of Large Language Models (LLMs), a hallucination does not mean the machine is seeing ghosts. It means the machine is confidently stating a fact that is entirely made up. Because these models are trained to be fluent and persuasive rather than truthful, they can fabricate medical studies, invent side effects, or misinterpret clinical guidelines with terrifying conviction. A chatbot might tell you to take a specific supplement dosage that is actually toxic, or cite a paper from a prestigious journal that does not exist.

This creates a perilous trap for the exhausted sleeper. When you are sleep deprived, your cognitive defences are down. You are desperate for a solution. If a smart, articulate AI tells you that a certain herbal combination is the cure, you are primed to believe it. The interface, often a friendly, conversational chat window, bypasses our scepticism in a way that a dry medical textbook never could.

The World Health Organization recognised this danger in its recent guidance on AI for health, explicitly calling out hallucinations as a core risk. The concern is not just that the AI will be wrong, but that it will be wrong in plausible ways. It might mix good advice with bad. It might correctly describe cognitive behavioural therapy for insomnia but then suggest a dangerous hack it learned from a dodgy Reddit forum in its training data.

Beyond pure fabrication, there is the problem of context blindness. A general purpose AI does not know your medical history unless you tell it, and even then, it may not understand the implications. For example, sleep restriction therapy is a standard, evidence based treatment for insomnia. It involves limiting time in bed to build sleep pressure. But for a person with bipolar disorder, sleep restriction can trigger a manic episode. A human clinician knows this red flag immediately. A chatbot, simply reciting a textbook protocol, might inadvertently push a vulnerable user into a mental health crisis.

This is why the distinction between wellness coaching and medical diagnosis is so critical, and yet so blurry in the world of AI. If an app tells you to drink less coffee, that is coaching. If it tells you that your breathing pattern suggests you have central sleep apnoea and you should buy a specific device, that is diagnosis. When AI crosses that line without regulatory oversight, patient safety is on the line.

Then there is the silent decay known as model drift. We tend to think of software as something that stays the same once it is installed. But AI models are organic in a sense; they live on data. A sleep model trained on a specific population say, healthy young men in a university study might perform incredibly well for that group. But apply that same model to a post-menopausal woman, or an elderly man with heart failure, and the predictions may fall apart.

Furthermore, the model can degrade over time as your own habits change. The algorithm that learned your sleep patterns when you were single and twenty five might be completely baffled by your sleep patterns now that you are thirty and have a newborn baby. If the model does not update its understanding of your baseline, it will start giving you advice for a person who no longer exists. It becomes a zombie pilot, flying by maps that are years out of date.

Hardware changes cause drift too. If the firmware on your smart watch updates and changes how it calculates heart rate variability, the AI model relying on that data might suddenly think you are stressed or sick, even if you are fine. This technical drift can lead to false alarms and unnecessary anxiety. It breaks the trust between the user and the co-pilot.

Bias is another ghost in the machine. AI models are only as good as the data they are fed. Historically, sleep science has suffered from a lack of diversity. Many foundational datasets are heavily skewed towards white, Western populations. If an AI model is trained on this biased data, it will bake that bias into its advice. It might systematically underestimate sleep apnoea risk in people with darker skin, or misinterpret the sleep architecture of non-Western populations. This is not just a technical glitch; it is an equity issue. It risks creating a two tiered system where the AI works perfectly for some and fails for others.

So, how do we navigate this minefield? The answer lies in guardrails and the human in the loop. Regulatory bodies are stepping in to demand that AI systems used for health meet higher standards of evidence. In the European Union and the United States, software that makes medical claims is increasingly treated as a medical device. This means it must undergo testing to prove it is safe and effective. It means the company cannot just release a beta version and hope for the best.

For the consumer, the best defence is a healthy scepticism. We should view generative AI as a powerful search engine and a tool for education, not as a doctor. It is excellent for summarising complex concepts, for helping you journal your sleep habits, or for suggesting general hygiene tips. It is terrible at diagnosing why you woke up gasping for air at 3am.

If your sleep app includes a chat assistant, treat it like a well-read friend who sometimes makes things up. Verify its claims. Check the sources. And most importantly, if you have a physical symptom such as a pause in breathing, a racing heart, chronic daytime sleepiness, do not ask the chatbot. Ask a clinician. The future of the AI co-pilot depends on solving these trust issues. We need models that know what they do not know. We need AI that can say, *I am not sure, please see a professional.* We need systems that are transparent about their training data and their limitations.

Until then, we must remember that fluency is not fact. The AI can write a beautiful sonnet about sleep, and it can generate a very convincing sleep schedule. But it does not sleep. It does not know what it feels like to be exhausted. It is a tool of immense potential, but it is one that requires a human hand on the wheel to keep it from driving us off the road. The risk of hallucination is the price of admission for this new technology, and vigilance is the only way to pay it.

The Future of Automated Environmental Control

The ultimate ambition of any good technology is to disappear. A light switch is technology, but you never think about it; you just flip it and the room changes. A thermostat is technology, but you rarely check the manual; you just turn the dial. The current generation of sleep technology has failed this test. It is loud, needy, and visible. It demands that you wear it, charge it, sync it, and look at it. It gives you homework. It tells you to lower the temperature or dim the lights, but it leaves the actual labour to you.

The final phase of the AI co-pilot is the move from advice to automation. This is the shift from an open loop system, where the human must intervene to close the circuit, to a closed loop system, where the machine senses a need and acts on it instantly and autonomously. We are entering the age of the automated bedroom.

In this future, the AI does not nag you to make the room cooler. It simply cools the room. It does not tell you that the lights are too bright for your current circadian phase. It simply dims them. The co-pilot stops being a coach standing on the sidelines shouting instructions and becomes the engineer running the ship while you rest.

The engine behind this shift is a branch of artificial intelligence called reinforcement learning. Unlike standard programming, where a human writes a rule like if it is 10pm, turn off the lights, reinforcement learning allows the system to learn by doing. The AI makes small adjustments to the environment and watches how your biology responds.

Imagine a smart bedroom hub that connects to your thermostat, your motorised blinds, your lighting, and your sleep tracker. On the first night, it might try lowering the temperature to eighteen degrees Celsius at 2am. It then checks your deep sleep data. If your deep sleep increases, the system gives itself a reward; a mathematical point for a good decision. If you wake up shivering or your sleep fragments, it gets a penalty. Over weeks and months, the system learns the unique thermal signature of your sleep. It learns that you need the room to be nineteen degrees when you first fall asleep, but that you run hot at 3am and need it to drop to seventeen, and then warm up slightly at 6am to help you wake. It learns that on days you exercise, you need a different profile than on days you are sedentary. It builds a dynamic, personalised control policy that no human could ever program manually (without running mad).

This applies to light as well. We know that the colour and intensity of light are critical for setting the body clock. An automated room can manage this spectrally. As the evening progresses, the system can slowly strip out the blue wavelengths from your smart bulbs, shifting the room to a warm amber glow that mimics a sunset. It can do this imperceptibly, shifting the colour temperature by a few kelvins every minute, so you never notice the change. You just find yourself naturally yawning at the right time.

In the morning, the reverse happens. The blinds can inch open precisely in sync with your sleep cycle. If the AI detects that you are in deep sleep ten minutes before your alarm, it might hold the blinds closed to let you finish the cycle. If it sees you are in light sleep, it might open them to flood the room with daylight, triggering the cortisol release that helps you wake up alert. The jarring sound of an alarm clock is replaced by the gentle physics of light.

Sound, too, enters the loop, and in an automated room, it becomes reactive. If a sensor on the window detects the frequency of a garbage truck coming down the street, the internal speakers can momentarily increase the volume of the masking pink noise to cover the spike. The room actively defends your sleep against the acoustic invasion of the city.

This level of automation sounds like science fiction, or perhaps a luxury hotel on Mars, but the components already exist. Smart thermostats, connected bulbs, and motorised shades are standard consumer goods. The missing piece has been the intelligence to coordinate them. We have had the instruments, but not the conductor. The AI co-pilot is that conductor.

However, for this future to be acceptable, it must be private. If your bedroom is constantly listening, watching, and adjusting, the privacy risks we discussed earlier become acute. This is why the industry is moving towards edge computing. This means that the AI processing happens locally, on a chip inside the device or the hub, rather than sending your data to a server in the cloud. In an edge-based system, your sleep data never leaves your house. The decision to lower the blinds is made by the computer on your nightstand, not by a server farm in another country. This privacy by design is non-negotiable for a technology that wants to live in our bedrooms. We will only invite the machine in if we know it cannot gossip about what it sees.

There is also a risk of fragility. A fully automated room is a complex system, and complex systems break. If the WiFi goes down, do the lights stay on? If the software crashes, does the heat turn off in winter? The engineering challenge is to build systems that fail safely and gracefully. The smart switch must still work as a dumb switch if the network fails. The technology must be robust enough to be ignored.

Ultimately, the future of automated environmental control is about returning to a simpler state of being. It is about using the most advanced technology humanity has ever created to replicate the most primitive environmental conditions: the cool, dark, quiet cave. We are using lasers, radar, and neural networks to give ourselves the same sleep experience our ancestors had for free.

It seems ironic, but it is necessary. We have built a world that is hostile to sleep; a world of constant light, noise, and stress. We cannot dismantle the modern world, so we must build micro-climates of sanctuary within it. The AI co-pilot allows us to carve out a space where biology still rules.

When this technology matures, the sleep economy will look very different. We will stop buying gadgets that tell us we are tired. We will start buying infrastructure that keeps us rested. We will stop obsessing over scores and start enjoying the silence. The best sleep technology of the future will be the one you never see, never touch, and never have to think about. It will just be a room that knows you, holds you, and lets you rest.

4

Rooms That Keep Time

> We shape our buildings, afterwards our buildings shape us.

WINSTON CHURCHILL

Light as a Drug

If you were to treat your bedroom not as a room, but as a terrarium for a rare and delicate species, you would approach its design very differently. You would not simply paint the walls a colour you liked and buy a comfortable rug. You would obsess over the environmental inputs. You would measure the humidity to the percentage point. You would ensure the temperature followed a precise gradient from day to night. And most importantly, you would control the light with absolute rigour, knowing that the wrong wavelength at the wrong time would damage the organism inside.

The reality is that you are that organism. Your bedroom is a biological containment unit, a biosphere that you seal yourself into for eight hours a day. And of all the environmental levers you can pull to support the biology inside that room, light is the undisputed master. It is the most potent drug we take, and we take it through our eyes.

For decades, we have misunderstood light. Architects and interior designers treated it as an aesthetic tool. They measured it in lux, a metric based on how bright a surface appears to the human visual system. If a room looked bright enough to read in, it was lit. But biology does not care about how a room looks; it cares about what time it is.

As briefly discussed in Chapter 1, deep inside the human eye, separate from the rods and cones that give us vision, lives a set of sensors called intrinsically photosensitive retinal ganglion cells (IPRG). These cells are not there to help you see the furniture. They are there to taste the sky. They are specifically tuned to detect blue-rich daylight. When they catch that signal, they send a direct message to the suprachiasmatic nucleus, the master clock in the brain, screaming that it is daytime. This triggers the release of cortisol for alertness and suppresses the release of melatonin.

This system works perfectly in the wild. But in the modern bedroom, it is often a disaster. We have flooded our nights with artificial light that mimics the sun. We stare into screens that pump blue photons directly into these ganglion cells at 10pm, effectively telling the brain that it is noon. We have uncoupled the light signal from the solar day.

The science of lighting has finally caught up to this problem. We have moved beyond vague terms like warm or cool white. We now have a precise standard called Melanopic Equivalent Daylight Illuminance, or Melanopic EDI. Think of this as the nutritional label for light. Just as we count calories for the body, we can now count melanopic lux for the brain. It measures how much a light source stimulates the circadian system, independent of how bright it looks.

This new metric gives us a prescription for the bedroom. The consensus from expert groups is that during the day, your eyes should receive a feast of light, at least 250 melanopic lux, to anchor your clock and boost your mood. But in the three hours before bed, that number needs to crash. You want no more than 10 melanopic lux. And while you are sleeping? You want zero. If you need a night light for safety, it should deliver no more than 1 melanopic lux.

This is the difference between a lighting scheme that looks nice and one that functions biologically. A standard LED bulb might look warm to the eye because it has a yellow tint, but it can still pump out enough blue energy to trigger your clock and suppress melatonin. A biological specification forces us to look at the spectral power distribution (the actual ingredients of the light) not just its colour.

There is a reason space agencies obsess over this. On the International Space Station, the sun rises and sets every ninety minutes. If astronauts relied on looking out the window to set their clocks, their circadian rhythms would shatter, leading to dangerous fatigue. To fix this, NASA replaced the old fluorescent modules on the station with a sophisticated, tuneable LED system.

This system is a dynamic drug delivery mechanism. When the crew needs to be alert for a docking procedure or a spacewalk, the lights shift to a high-intensity, blue-enriched spectrum that forces the brain into wakefulness. When it is time for the pre-sleep period, the blue drops out entirely, shifting to a sleepy, low-intensity red. If we can entrain a human body clock while it is hurling through the vacuum of space at seventeen thousand miles per hour, we can certainly do it in a semi-detached house in the suburbs.

We are seeing this logic move from orbit to the ward. Hospitals are notoriously bad places to sleep. They are bright, loud, and run on a 24-hour cycle that ignores the sun. But new circadian lighting trials in cardiology units and ICUs are changing the game. By programming the ward lights to mimic the solar day, i.e. bright and blue in the morning, dim and warm in the evening, hospitals can stabilise patient sleep patterns. Early data suggests this can improve sleep duration and perhaps even speed up recovery. It turns out that when you stop fighting the patient's body clock, the body heals better.

So, how does this translate to your programmable sanctuary? It means you need to stop thinking about lights on and lights off and start thinking about scenes.

Your bedroom needs a morning scene. This is a blast of light. If you have smart blinds, they should open automatically at your wake time. If you live in a dark apartment, you might need a dawn simulator or a high-quality light box or AI enabled lamp, that delivers that critical 250 melanopic lux while you get dressed. This signal tells your brain to dump the last of the melatonin and start the timer for tonight's sleep. The clock starts ticking the moment the light hits your retina.

Then, you need an evening scene. This is where most homes fail. We leave the big overhead light on while we brush our teeth and pack our bags. That single blast of bright, overhead light is a dose of anti-sleep drug. The evening scene should rely on lamps placed below eye level. The light should be amber or red-shifted. It should be dim - dimmer than you think. You need just enough light to navigate safely, not enough to simulate the sun.

Finally, you need a darkness protocol. We are incredibly sensitive to light at night. Even a small amount of light leaking in from a streetlamp, or the standby LED on a television, can impact sleep structure. One laboratory study showed that sleeping with a modest room light (about 100 lux) was enough to raise heart rate and mess with insulin sensitivity by the next morning. Your body detects the light even through closed eyelids.

This means blackout curtains are not an aesthetic choice; they are a health intervention. It means covering the LEDs on your air purifier with tape. It means that if you get up to use the bathroom, you do not flip the main switch. You use a tiny, motion-activated nightlight that stays low to the ground and emits a soft amber glow. You navigate by moon-mode, not sun-mode.

The beauty of this approach is that once you set it up, you can ignore it. You do not need willpower to lower your melatonin suppression; you just need a timer on your smart bulb. You do not need to remind yourself to wake up; the light does it for you.

We often talk about blue light as the villain, blaming our phones and tablets. And while staring at a screen is bad, the ambient light in the room is often the bigger culprit simply because of the dosage. The photon bomb of a kitchen down-light while you get a glass of water is a far stronger signal than the glow of a kindle on its lowest setting.

We are moving towards a future where 'circadian safe' will be a standard feature of building codes, just like fire safety. Architects will specify melanopic EDI targets for evening living spaces. Windows will tint automatically to balance daylight. But until that future arrives, you have to be the lighting engineer of your own life.

Treat light with the respect you would give a prescription medication. Take a high dose in the morning. Taper the dose in the evening. And avoid it completely at night. If you get the light right, the biology tends to follow. The terrarium is set; the organism can finally rest.

The Soundscape of Recovery

If light is the master clock signal that tells the brain when to sleep, sound is the sentry that decides if it is safe to stay asleep. For millions of years, our auditory system has evolved to be the primary alarm system of the night. While our eyelids close to shut out the visual world, our ears have no lids. They remain open, processing every vibration in the air, filtering the signal from the noise, and standing guard against the snap of a twig that might signal a predator.

In the modern world, the predators are gone, but the noise remains. In fact, the acoustic environment of the twenty-first-century city is a chaotic barrage of signals that our ancient biology is ill-equipped to handle. We have replaced the snap of a twig with the roar of a motorbike, the wail of a siren, and the low-frequency rumble of a passing bus. We are trying to sleep in a sonic war zone.

The second lever in your programmable sanctuary is the soundscape. Managing it is not just about making the room quiet. It is about smoothing the edges of the world outside. The problem with sound during sleep is rarely the absolute volume. It is the sudden change. The brain is an expert at habituation. It can get used to the steady hum of an air conditioner or the rhythmic woosh of the ocean. It can label those sounds as safe background data and ignore them.

What the brain cannot ignore is the spike. A single motorbike accelerating at 2am can be far more disruptive than a constant stream of highway traffic. The sudden shift in decibels triggers an arousal response. Your heart rate spikes, your blood pressure rises, and your brain shifts from deep, restorative sleep into lighter stages or full wakefulness. You might not even remember waking up, but the damage to your sleep architecture is done. You wake up tired, the victim of a hundred micro-arousals you never consciously registered.

This is a public health issue. The World Health Organization has established strict guidelines for night noise, recommending that outdoor noise levels should remain below forty to forty-five decibels to protect public health. Exposure above these levels is linked not just to annoyance, but to vascular stress and a higher risk of hypertension. When your bedroom is loud, your cardiovascular system stays on alert all night. You are resting, but your heart is not.

Since we cannot rebuild our cities or silence our neighbours, we must engineer the room to handle the intrusion. The most effective tool for this is acoustic masking. This is often confused with noise cancellation, but the physics are different. Active noise cancellation, like the kind found in expensive headphones, listens to the world and produces an anti-wave to erase the sound. That works well for the drone of an aeroplane engine, but it is hard to do in a three-dimensional room without wearing a headset.

Masking takes a different approach. Instead of erasing the noise, it buries it. By introducing a steady, broadband sound into the room, you raise the acoustic floor. This reduces the dynamic range between the background silence and the sudden intrusion. If your room is dead silent at twenty decibels, a sixty-decibel truck is a massive shock. If your room is humming along at forty decibels of steady masking sound, that same truck is only a twenty-decibel ripple. The spike is flattened. The sentry in your brain stays calm.

This is the science behind white noise, but true white noise, which sounds like harsh static, is often too high-pitched for comfort. Most sleep engineers prefer pink noise or brown noise. Pink noise is balanced so that every octave carries equal energy, sounding more like heavy rain or wind in the trees. Brown noise is even deeper, a low rumble like a distant waterfall or thunder. These sounds are biologically soothing because they mask the sharp frequencies of human speech and traffic without being abrasive themselves.

There is a more advanced frontier here as well. Researchers are experimenting with closed-loop auditory stimulation. This involves a system that listens to your brain waves via a headband. When it detects the slow, rhythmic pulses of deep sleep, it plays a tiny burst of pink noise at the exact millisecond the brain wave is rising. This audio nudge acts like a push on a swing, amplifying the brain wave and deepening the sleep state. In lab studies, this has been shown to boost memory consolidation and restorative sleep. While consumer versions are still maturing, the principle proves that sound can be more than a shield. It can be a performance enhancer.

For the practical programmable room, the solution is often low-tech. A mechanical fan is one of the best sleep devices ever invented. It provides a steady, non-looping airflow sound that covers a wide range of frequencies. It is the original brown noise machine. For those who need more control, electronic sound machines can generate precise acoustic curtains. The key is to keep the volume low and the sound constant.

The one sound that has no place in the recovery landscape is the television. Many people rely on the TV to fall asleep, using it as a distraction from racing thoughts. But the television is an acoustic rollercoaster. It has dialogue, explosions, music swells, and sudden silences. It is designed to capture attention, not release it. The flickering light and the variable sound keep the brain in a state of shallow engagement. If you need a voice to soothe you, choose a monotone podcast or a sleep story designed to be boring, and put it on a timer so the silence eventually takes over.

We must also consider the silence itself. In a well-engineered room, silence is the canvas. Heavy curtains do not just block light; they dampen sound reflections. Soft furnishings, rugs, and upholstered headboards absorb the high-frequency echoes that make a room feel brittle and loud. Sealing the gaps around the door with a simple draft stopper can cut the noise transfer from the rest of the house significantly.

The goal is to build a sonic cocoon. You want to create an environment where the auditory horizon shrinks to the four walls of your room. When the soundscape is steady and safe, the brain's sentinel can finally stand down. It stops scanning for threats and allows the mind to descend into the deep, unprotected states of recovery that we so desperately need. In the programmable sanctuary, peace and quiet is not just a luxury. It is an engineering specification.

Thermal Engineering

If light is the master clock of the sleep system, temperature is the steering wheel. We often think of feeling hot or cold as a comfort issue, a matter of personal preference like firm or soft pillows. But biologically, temperature is a control signal. It is the physical mechanism the body uses to initiate and maintain the state of sleep. To fall asleep, your core body temperature must drop. To stay asleep, it must stay low. And to wake up, it must rise again.

The programmable sanctuary must therefore be a thermal engine. It needs to facilitate this shedding of heat in the evening and protect the sleeper from overheating in the night. This is not just about setting a thermostat to a magic number; it is about managing the microclimate that exists between your skin and the mattress.

The physiology is elegant. As evening approaches and melatonin rises, the body prepares to cool down. It does this by opening up the blood vessels in the hands and feet, a process called vasodilation. This sends warm blood away from the core to the surface of the skin, where the heat can radiate out into the room. This is why a warm bath or shower before bed is such a powerful sleep hack. It seems counterintuitive to heat up to cool down, but the hot water triggers a massive vasodilation event. When you step out of the bath into the cooler air of the bedroom, the heat dumps rapidly from your skin, driving your core temperature down and signalling to the brain that it is time to sleep.

However, once you are in bed, the challenge changes. You are now sandwiched between an insulating mattress and an insulating duvet. If the room is too warm, or the bedding is not breathable, that heat has nowhere to go. It gets trapped next to the skin. This is the thermal trap of the modern bedroom. Memory foam mattresses, while excellent for pressure relief, are notorious heat sinks. They absorb body heat and hold it, slowly baking the sleeper as the night progresses.

When the body gets too hot, it has to fight back. It increases heart rate. It sweats. It shifts into a lighter stage of sleep or wakes you up entirely to throw off the covers. This is why a hot room is the enemy of deep sleep. Studies suggest that for most adults, the ideal ambient temperature for sleep is surprisingly cool, often between 18 and 20 degrees Celsius. This ambient chill allows the head, which remains exposed, to dissipate heat effectively while the body stays cozy under the covers. For older people the room should really be under 24 degrees Celsius to prevent heat-stress and exhaustion risks.

But setting the whole house to 18 degrees Celsius is expensive and sometimes uncomfortable for partners who run at different temperatures. This is where thermal engineering at the level of the bed becomes transformative. We are seeing a boom in active cooling technologies. These are mattress covers and pads that circulate water or air through thin channels. They act like a radiator for the bed, pulling heat away from the body and dumping it elsewhere.

The most advanced of these systems are programmable. They can set a thermal profile for the night. You might start with a warm bed to help you get cozy and relax. Then, as you fall asleep, the system ramps down the temperature to support the deep sleep phase, which is most sensitive to heat. Finally, in the early morning, it gently warms the bed to trigger the wake-up signal, mimicking the rising sun. This dynamic control aligns the environment with the biological need, rather than forcing the biology to adapt to a static room.

For perimenopausal and menopausal women, this technology is not just a luxury; it is a lifeline. Hot flashes and night sweats are profound disruptors of sleep. They are surges of heat that can wake a woman from a dead sleep, drenched and adrenaline-filled. Active cooling provides a way to manage this that no amount of willpower can achieve. By keeping the bed surface cool, the system can blunt the intensity of the flash and help the sleeper return to unconsciousness faster.

Passive tools play a role too. Phase change materials are now being woven into sheets and pyjamas. These are smart fabrics that absorb heat when you get too hot and release it when you cool down, acting as a thermal buffer. They smooth out the peaks and troughs of the night. Even the humble fan is a hero here. Gentle airflow across the body increases evaporative cooling, allowing you to sleep comfortably in a warmer room without the noise and expense of air conditioning.

The goal of thermal engineering is to uncouple the sleeper from the weather. It is to create a stable, neutral thermal environment where the body's own thermoregulation systems can work without strain. When the bed handles the heat, the heart can slow down, the sweat glands can rest, and the brain can stay deep in the delta waves of recovery. In the programmable sanctuary, being cool is not just a state of mind; it is a biological necessity.

The Invisible Atmosphere

You can perfect the lighting, soundproof the walls, and cool the bed to a precise nineteen degrees, and still wake up feeling groggy and unrefreshed. The culprit in this scenario is often the one element we cannot see and rarely think about: the air itself.

We tend to treat the air in our bedrooms as a constant, assuming that as long as we can breathe, the air is working. But biologically, the composition of that air changes dramatically over the course of the night, and those changes can have a profound impact on the quality of our rest. The programmable sanctuary must account for the invisible atmosphere.

The primary enemy of the sealed bedroom is carbon dioxide (CO_2). We are used to thinking of CO_2 as a global climate issue, but it is also a microclimate issue. When you enter your bedroom at 10pm, the CO_2 levels are likely close to the ambient outdoor level, roughly 400 to 500 parts per million (ppm). But modern homes are built to be energy efficient. We seal them tight with double glazing and insulation to keep the heat (or the cool) in.

When you close the door and windows to sleep, you create a sealed capsule. As you breathe, you inhale oxygen and exhale carbon dioxide. Over the course of eight hours, two adults and a large dog sleeping in a small, sealed room can easily drive the CO_2 levels up to 2500 or 3000 ppm.

While these levels are not toxic in the sense that they will kill you, they are physiologically significant. Research into indoor air quality has shown that as CO_2 rises above 1000 ppm, cognitive function begins to decline. In the context of sleep, high CO_2 levels have been linked to an increase in arousals, a decrease in deep sleep, and that specific, heavy-headed feeling of stuffiness upon waking. You wake up feeling like you have a mild hangover, not because you drank alcohol, but because you spent the night breathing your own exhaust fumes.

The solution in the programmable room is active ventilation. In a sophisticated smart home, a CO_2 sensor on the bedside table acts as the trigger. When levels climb past 800 ppm, it sends a signal to the HVAC system to cycle fresh air from outside, or even to a motorised window actuator to crack the window open by an inch. The goal is to keep the bedroom biosphere as close to fresh outdoor air as possible, maintaining the oxygen richness required for the brain's nightly repair work.

The second variable is particulate matter. The bedroom is often the dustiest room in the house, filled with shedding skin cells, dust mites, and fabric fibres from bedding. If you live in a city, you are also battling pollution from traffic, pollen, and smoke. When we sleep, our airways relax. If the air is thick with irritants, the body fights back with inflammation. The nasal passages swell, increasing resistance to breathing. This can turn a silent sleeper into a snorer, or push a mild snorer into sleep apnoea.

An air purifier is therefore not just a gadget for allergy sufferers; it is a piece of sleep infrastructure. A high-quality HEPA filter running quietly in the corner scrubs the air of these microscopic agitators. It reduces the inflammatory load on the respiratory system. By keeping the nose clear, it promotes nasal breathing, which is crucial for maintaining the correct balance of oxygen and nitric oxide in the blood.

Finally, we must manage humidity. This is the Goldilocks variable. If the air is too dry (which is common in winter with central heating) the mucous membranes of the nose and throat dry out. They become irritated and sticky, increasing the risk of infection and snoring. If the air is too humid, it becomes heavy and difficult to cool, preventing the sweat evaporation that helps lower body temperature. High humidity also encourages the growth of mould and dust mites.

The programmable room aims for the neutral zone, typically between 40 and 60 per cent relative humidity. Smart humidifiers can add moisture when the heating is on, and the air conditioning or a dehumidifier can strip it out during a muggy summer night.

This attention to the invisible atmosphere is the final step in creating a sleep tank. It acknowledges that sleep is a metabolic process. It requires fuel (oxygen) and it produces waste (CO_2). If we do not engineer the room to manage this exchange, we are limiting the efficiency of our recovery. We spend a third of our lives in this one room. Ensuring the air we breathe there is as pure as a mountain top is one of the highest yield investments we can make in our health.

The Integrated Audit

We have looked at the four pillars of the programmable sanctuary: light, sound, temperature, and air. Treated in isolation, each one is a powerful lever for better sleep. But a bedroom is not a series of isolated variables. It is a system. The light affects the temperature. The airflow affects the sound. To truly engineer a space for recovery, we need to look at how these elements integrate. We need to stop seeing the bedroom as a collection of furniture and start seeing it as a performance envelope.

The best way to do this is to perform a sensory audit. This is a practical, ten-minute process that you can do tonight. It requires no expensive equipment, just your own senses and a critical mindset. It involves walking into your room not as a tired person looking for a bed, but as an engineer looking for friction.

Start with the light audit. Turn off every light in the room and close the door. Stand in the centre of the room and wait for two minutes to let your eyes adjust to the darkness. Now, look around. What do you see? In most modern bedrooms, you will see a constellation of artificial stars. The standby light on the television. The charging LED on the vacuum cleaner in the corner. The green glow of the smoke alarm. The light leaking in from the streetlamp through the gap in the curtains.

Each of these is a signal leak. Each one is a photon intruder. The fix is often low-tech. A roll of black electrical tape is one of the most effective sleep tools you can buy. Tape over the LEDs. Buy blocking strips to seal the gaps in your blinds. Your goal is a room so dark that you cannot see your hand in front of your face. This absolute darkness signals to the brain that the solar day is unequivocally over.

Next, do the sound audit. Close your eyes and listen. What is the baseline noise floor of the room? Is it dead silent, so silent that a floorboard creaking sounds like a gunshot? Or is there a chaotic mix of traffic and house noise? If it is too quiet, you need to raise the floor with acoustic masking, i.e. a fan or a sound machine. If it is too loud, you need to dampen the room. Look at the hard surfaces. Can you add a rug? Can you hang heavier curtains? Can you move the bed away from the shared wall? You are trying to build a sonic buffer that protects the brain from sudden spikes.

Then, check the thermal environment. Put your hand on your mattress. Is it warm to the touch? If it feels warm now, it will be a furnace in four hours. Consider the materials. If you are sleeping on synthetic sheets and a foam block, you are wrapping yourself in plastic insulation. Look for breathable, natural fibres like cotton, bamboo, or wool. Check the airflow. Is the air stagnant? A simple fan moving air across the bed can lower the effective temperature by several degrees through the wind-chill effect, without the cost of air conditioning.

Finally, assess the air. Walk out of the room, close the door, and come back in after ten minutes. Does the room smell stuffy or stale compared to the hallway? That is the smell of CO_2 and trapped humidity. If you detect it, you need ventilation. Even opening the window a crack, or leaving the bedroom door slightly ajar, can create enough cross-breeze to flush the room of stale air.

To see how this comes together in the real world, consider the case of a shift worker living on the Gold Coast. This is an extreme environment for sleep: high heat, high humidity, and bright tropical sun, combined with a schedule that demands sleep at 11am. For this sleeper, the integrated audit leads to a bunker strategy. The light is managed not just with curtains, but with aluminium foil taped directly to the glass to reflect 100 per cent of the sun. The sound is managed with heavy-duty earplugs and a loud, industrial fan that drowns out the daytime traffic. The temperature is managed by blasting the air conditioning for an hour before bed to super-cool the mattress, then setting it to a maintenance level. It is an aggressive, engineered environment, but it allows biology to function against the grain of the solar day.

Contrast this with a couple in London during winter. Their challenge is different. One partner freezes; the other burns up. Their integrated audit focuses on the microclimate of the bed. They might use the Scandinavian method of two separate duvets, allowing the cold sleeper to have a heavy tog rating and the hot sleeper to use a light sheet. They might use an active cooling pad on just one side of the bed. They keep the window cracked for fresh air (low CO_2) but use a heated throw rug to warm the bed before getting in.

These examples show that there is no single perfect room. There is only the room that solves your specific problems. The programmable sanctuary is adaptable. It changes with the seasons, with your age, and with your life circumstances. The shift from the static bedroom to the programmable sanctuary is the final piece of the puzzle. We have discussed the sensors that measure us (Chapter 1 & 2), the AI that guides us (Chapter 3), and now the environment that holds us (Chapter 4).

When you align these three layers, the measured body, the intelligent insight, and the engineered space, you create the conditions for a sleep revolution.

You stop fighting your biology and start supporting it. You stop wondering why you are tired and start understanding the inputs that lead to recovery. The room becomes a machine for rest, a silent partner in your health. And the best part? Once you have engineered it, you can stop thinking about it. You can just close your eyes, safe in the knowledge that the darkness, the silence, and the cool air are all working in concert to carry you through the night.

5

Sleep Clinic In The Bedroom

Medicine is a science of uncertainty & an art of probability.

SIR WILLIAM OSLER

The Decentralised Clinical Lab

For nearly half a century, the only way to truly understand what was happening to a human being during sleep was to remove them from their natural habitat. If you suspected you had a sleep disorder, you were referred to a hospital or a specialised clinic. You would arrive in the evening, be shown to a sterile room that tried and failed to look like a hotel, and then spend an hour having electrodes glued to your scalp, face, chest, and legs. You would be wrapped in belts, cannulas, and wires, and then told to sleep naturally while a technician watched you via an infrared camera from the room next door.

This process, known as polysomnography, remains the gold standard of diagnostic medicine. It is incredibly detailed, capturing every electrical whisper of the brain and every twitch of the muscle. But it has a fundamental flaw: it is deeply artificial. The very act of measuring the sleep changes the sleep. This is known in the industry as the first night effect, where the anxiety and discomfort of the environment cause the patient to sleep far worse than they normally would, potentially skewing the data. Furthermore, these labs are expensive, labour intensive, and scarce. In many public health systems, the waiting list for a sleep study can stretch to months or even years.

We are now witnessing the dismantling of this bottleneck. We are moving from the centralised model of the hospital to the decentralised model of the bedroom. The clinic is coming to you. The primary driver of this shift is the Home Sleep Apnoea Test (HSAT). These devices have stripped the diagnostic process down to its essentials. Instead of a cart full of equipment, the patient receives a small kit in the mail, about the size of a lunchbox. Inside is a simplified sensor array: a clip for the finger to measure oxygen and heart rate, a belt for the chest to measure respiratory effort, and a cannula for the nose to measure airflow.

The patient puts it on themselves before bed, sleeps in their own room, in their own temperature settings, with their own pillows and bedding. The device records the night's data to a memory card or uploads it directly to the cloud. In the morning, they put it back in the box and post it back. This shift is not just about comfort; it is about scale. Obstructive sleep apnoea is a pandemic of the modern age, affecting an estimated one billion people globally, yet nearly eighty per cent of cases remain undiagnosed. There are simply not enough hospital beds in the world to test everyone who needs testing. The decentralised clinic solves this logistics problem. It allows a single sleep physician to diagnose thousands of patients remotely, rather than hundreds in person.

It also changes the demographic of who gets treated. In the old model, you had to be sick enough to justify a night in hospital. In the new model, the barrier to entry is low. If you are feeling tired or your partner says you snore, you can order a test online or pick one up from a pharmacy. This early detection is crucial. It catches the disease in the mild to moderate stage, before it has had decades to ravage the cardiovascular system and affect the brain.

However, the decentralised clinic requires a new kind of literacy. The patient is no longer a passive subject; they are also a technician. They have to apply the sensors correctly. They have to ensure the WiFi is connected. While the devices are designed to be idiot proof, with flashing lights and voice prompts, human error is still a variable. A loose belt or a slipped cannula can result in a night of useless data, requiring a retest.

Furthermore, these home devices generally focus almost exclusively on breathing and oxygen, most do not record EEG (brain waves). This means they cannot technically tell if you are asleep or awake; they just assume you are asleep during the recording period. For a patient with severe sleep apnoea, this doesn't matter much as the breathing pauses are obvious. But for a patient with insomnia or a complex neurological issue, the home test might miss the mark completely.

Despite these limitations, the trajectory is irreversible. The technology is getting smaller and smarter. We are seeing disposable, single use test kits that look like a simple plaster on the wrist. We are seeing the integration of these medical diagnostics into consumer wearables, blurring the line between a smartwatch and a medical device.

The decentralised clinic represents a fundamental change in the power dynamic of medicine. It respects the patient's time and environment. It acknowledges that sleep is an intimate act that is best measured in private. By moving the diagnostic front line into the bedroom, we are finally treating sleep disorders where they actually happen, rather than where the machines happen to be kept.

Therapeutic Evolution

For decades, the diagnosis of sleep apnoea led almost inevitably to a single destination: the CPAP machine. Continuous Positive Airway Pressure was, and remains, a medical miracle. Invented in the early 1980s using a vacuum cleaner motor and some tubing, it works on a principle of pneumatic splinting. By blowing a stream of air down the throat, it creates enough pressure to hold the collapsing tissues open, allowing the patient to breathe freely. It is 100 per cent effective if used correctly.

The problem, of course, is the *if*. For many patients, being tethered to a bedside turbine via a plastic hose and a face mask is a claustrophobic nightmare. The adherence rates for CPAP have historically been poor, with roughly half of all patients abandoning the therapy within the first year. This resistance has driven a rapid evolution in therapeutic hardware. We are moving away from the Darth Vader aesthetic of the early days towards a design philosophy that prioritises minimalism and comfort. The goal is to make the medical equipment feel less medical.

The first frontier of this evolution is the interface: the mask itself. Early masks were heavy, industrial rubber triangles that covered the nose and mouth, strapped tight to the face to prevent leaks. Today, we have nasal pillows and nasal cradles that sit gently under the nostrils, secured by minimalist silicone headgear. They are quiet, lightweight, and designed to allow the user to read or wear glasses in bed. The use of magnetic clips allows users to snap the mask on and off in the dark without fumbling with Velcro. These seem like small tweaks, but in the context of a therapy you have to use every single night for the rest of your life, friction reduction is everything.

However, the most significant shift is the realisation that not everyone needs a machine. We are seeing a boom in oral appliance therapy. These are custom-made devices, fabricated by specialist dentists, that look like a heavy-duty sports mouthguard. They work on a mechanical principle known as mandibular advancement. By clipping over the upper and lower teeth, the device holds the lower jaw in a forward position during sleep. This pulls the tongue forward and tightens the soft tissues of the throat, mechanically enlarging the airway. They are silent, portable, and require no electricity.

Then there is the role of gravity. For a significant percentage of patients, their apnoea is positional. Their airway only collapses when they sleep on their back, where gravity pulls the tongue and soft palate directly backward. When they sleep on their side, they are essentially cured. In the past, the low-tech solution for this was to sew a tennis ball into the back of a t-shirt. Today, we have electronic positional therapy. These are small, wearable devices worn on the chest or neck. They contain an accelerometer that knows the body's orientation. If the patient rolls onto their back, the device delivers a gentle vibration; not enough to wake them up fully, but enough to annoy them into rolling over. It is a form of Pavlovian conditioning for sleep posture as it turns the body's position into the therapy itself.

We are also seeing the emergence of expiratory positive airway pressure (EPAP) valves. These are tiny, disposable adhesive valves that stick over the nostrils. They allow air to flow in freely, but create resistance when you breathe out. This back-pressure keeps the airway inflated during the exhalation phase of the breath cycle. It is essentially a CPAP machine without the machine, powered by the patient's own lungs. The trajectory of this therapeutic evolution is towards personalisation. We are moving away from a one-size-fits-all model where everyone gets the same blower and the same pressure. We are entering an era of phenotyping, where a clinician looks at the specific anatomy and physiology of the collapse: is it the tongue? Is it the palate? Is it position-dependent? They then select the tool that fits the mechanism.

The bedroom is no longer just a place for a machine; it is a space for a toolkit. Whether it is a magnetised mask, a 3D-printed dental splint, or a vibrating chest strap, the focus has shifted from simply keeping the airway open to keeping the patient on board. Medicine in the bedroom only works if it can coexist with the life in the bedroom.

Pharmacology and Physiology

For the last forty years, sleep medicine has been dominated by physics. The problem of obstructive sleep apnoea was viewed as a mechanical failure: a tube (the throat) was collapsing under pressure (weight), and the solution was to prop it open with a pneumatic splint (CPAP). It was a plumbing solution to a biological problem.

But in the last few years, the ground has shifted beneath the field. We have entered the era of chemistry. The arrival of a new class of drugs known as glucagon-like peptide-1 (GLP-1) agonists, sold under brand names like Ozempic, Wegovy, and Mounjaro, is not just transforming the treatment of diabetes and obesity; it is fundamentally altering the landscape of sleep medicine.

To understand why, we have to look at the anatomy of the collapse. While sleep apnoea can occur in thin people due to jaw structure or genetics, the single biggest risk factor is excess weight. Specifically, visceral fat stored around the neck and in the tongue creates an anatomical crush. It narrows the airway and adds weight to the soft tissues, making them far more likely to collapse when muscle tone drops during sleep.

Historically, doctors told patients to lose weight as a first-line treatment. But sustainable weight loss is notoriously difficult, and sleep deprivation makes it harder by disrupting hunger hormones (ghrelin and leptin). It was a vicious cycle: the patient was too tired to exercise and too hormonally dysregulated to diet, so they gained more weight, which made the apnoea worse, which made them more tired.

GLP-1s break this cycle. By mimicking the hormone that signals satiety to the brain and slowing gastric emptying, these drugs drive profound weight loss; often fifteen to twenty per cent of body weight. When that weight comes off, it comes off the neck and the tongue, effectively de-crowding the airway.

Recent trials focusing specifically on patients with obstructive sleep apnoea have shown that these drugs can significantly reduce the Apnoea-Hypopnoea Index (AHI) which is the score that measures the severity of the disease. For some patients, the reduction is dramatic enough to move them from severe to mild, or even into remission.

This introduces a radical new possibility: deprescribing. Until now, a CPAP prescription was a life sentence because you were told you would wear the mask every night forever. Now, we are looking at a future where a patient might use CPAP as a bridge therapy while the pharmacology does the heavy lifting. Once the weight is down and the airway mechanics improve, the machine might go back in the closet.

There is also emerging interest in whether these drugs have benefits beyond simple mass/weight reduction. Obesity is an inflammatory state, and inflammation in the upper airway makes the tissues swollen and sticky, prone to collapse. By reducing systemic inflammation, GLP-1s might be improving airway compliance through a second, chemical pathway. However, this is not a magic bullet without consequences. These are powerful drugs with potential side effects and there is also the question of cost and access, and critically, apnoea is multifactorial. If your apnoea is driven by a receding chin or large tonsils, losing twenty kilos will help, but it will not cure you. The drug treats the anatomy of fat, not the anatomy of bone.

Despite all these caveats, the paradigm has shifted. Sleep medicine is moving from a discipline of air to a discipline of air and molecules. The bedroom of the future might not just contain a mask on the nightstand, but a weekly injection in the fridge.

We are finally treating the root cause, the physiological burden on the airway, rather than just managing the symptom of the collapse. The best machine for keeping the airway open might turn out not to be a machine at all, but a healthier metabolism.

Remote Patient Monitoring

The modern bedroom is no longer a private island. It has been connected to the mainland of the medical system by an invisible digital umbilical cord. In the past, when a patient was prescribed a therapy for a chronic condition, they were essentially sent out into the wilderness. They would leave the clinic with a device or a prescription, and the doctor would not know if they were using it, or if it was working, until the patient returned for a follow-up appointment six months later. During that long interval of silence, problems would fester. Masks would leak, pressures would feel suffocating, and motivation would evaporate. The therapy would fail in the dark.

Today, that silence has been filled with data. We have entered the age of Remote Patient Monitoring (RPM), a paradigm shift that turns the home bedroom into a satellite ward of the hospital. This is not a future prediction; it is the current reality for millions of people. Every night, as they sleep, their bedside devices are quietly talking to the cloud, transmitting a detailed dossier of their biological performance to a server farm, which then relays it to a clinical dashboard hundreds of kilometres away.

The technology driving this is the cellular modem. Almost every modern CPAP machine and high-end home ventilator now comes with a built-in transmission chip, similar to the one in your smartphone. It does not require the patient to pair it with WiFi or wrestle with Bluetooth settings. It just works. Minutes after the patient takes off their mask in the morning, the machine automatically phones home. It sends a packet of data containing the hours of use, the seal of the mask, the residual number of apnoea events, and the pressure profile of the night.

For the clinician, this transforms the practice of medicine from reactive to proactive. In the old model, a sleep technician would spend their day wading through the files of stable patients who were doing fine, potentially missing the crisis developing in a patient who didn't call. In the RPM model, the software acts as a triage nurse. It uses exception management algorithms to filter the population.

Imagine a dashboard on a computer screen. It displays a list of five thousand patients and four thousand nine hundred of them are marked with a green dot. The software has analysed their nightly data and confirmed they are using the therapy for more than four hours, their mask seal is perfect, and their therapy is effectively treating the apnoea. The clinician does not need to look at these files. They can focus their entire attention on the one hundred red dots as these are the patients who are struggling.

This ability to spot the strugglers in near real-time is the superpower of RPM. Consider a new patient, let's call him John, who is struggling with his new mask. On his third night of therapy, he rips the mask off at 2am because the pressure feels too high and the air is leaking into his eyes. In the old world, John would wake up angry, throw the machine in the closet, and give up. He might not tell his doctor for months.

In the RPM world, John's red dot appears on the technician's screen the next morning. The data shows a massive leak spike at 1:45am followed by a usage cessation at 2am. The technician can see exactly what happened without John saying a word. They can pick up the phone and call him. *"Hi John, I see you had a rough night around 2am. It looks like the mask shifted and the pressure ramped up. Let's adjust the settings together"*.

Crucially, this adjustment can often be done over the air. The clinician can log into the portal, change the pressure settings or the humidity level on the digital prescription, and beam the new instructions directly to John's bedside table. When John goes to bed that night, the machine has already been updated. The problem is solved without a clinic visit, without any significant cost, and without the patient losing faith in the therapy. This loop of detect, contact, adjust, is the heartbeat of modern adherence management.

However, this constant surveillance introduces a complex psychological dynamic. It brings the medical gaze into the most intimate space in the house. Patients know they are being watched. For some, this is a comfort; they feel supported and safe, knowing a safety net is spread beneath them. For others, it creates a sense of performance anxiety. Sleep, which should be an act of surrender, becomes an act of compliance.

This is particularly acute in healthcare systems where reimbursement is tied to usage. In the United States, for example, insurance companies often operate on a use it or lose it basis. They monitor the cloud data to ensure the patient is using the machine for a minimum number of hours (usually four hours a night for 70 per cent of nights). If the data shows non-compliance, the insurer may refuse to pay for the device or the supplies. Here, the modem is not just a clinical tool; it is an auditor. It turns the bedroom into a site of financial verification.

Similarly, for commercial truck drivers or train operators, this data is a condition of employment. Their licence to work depends on proving to the transport authority that their sleep apnoea is being treated. The Big Brother aspect of RPM is undeniable in these high-stakes scenarios. The machine that helps them breathe is also the machine that reports them if they fail to follow protocol.

Despite these tensions, the clinical benefits are overwhelming. Big Data studies analysing millions of nights of patient data have shown that engagement with RPM platforms significantly boosts long-term adherence. When patients have access to their own data, via a companion app on their phone that gives them a sleep score and coaching tips, they become active participants in their care. They start to gamify their own therapy. They want to get that 100 score or they want to fix their own leak. The data empowers them to own the problem.

The future of RPM is to move beyond the single channel of the CPAP machine. The bedroom is filling up with other sensors, e.g. connected blood pressure cuffs, smart scales, oxygen saturation rings. The goal is to integrate these disparate streams into a holistic view of the patient's health. We are moving towards a multi-parametric monitoring system. The clinician of the future won't just see that your apnoea is treated; they will see that on the nights you used your CPAP, your blood pressure dropped by five points the next morning, and your heart rate variability improved. They will be able to correlate the quality of your sleep with the stability of your heart failure or the management of your diabetes.

This allows for the management of comorbidities in a way that was never possible before. Sleep apnoea rarely travels alone; it brings friends like hypertension, atrial fibrillation, and Type 2 diabetes. RPM allows the care team to see the interplay between these conditions. If a patient with heart failure suddenly starts having 'Cheyne-Stokes' respiration (a specific, rhythmic breathing pattern detectable by the machine), the sleep data acts as an early warning system for the cardiologist. The bedroom sensor detects the decompensation of the heart days before the patient feels the fluid in their lungs.

Ultimately, Remote Patient Monitoring redefines the geography of the hospital. It dissolves the walls of the clinic. It acknowledges that chronic disease is lived twenty-four hours a day, not just during a fifteen-minute rushed consultation. By keeping a digital eye on the sleeper, the medical system can offer a level of continuity and safety that was previously the domain of the Intensive Care Unit. It is a profound trade-off: we give up a degree of privacy in our bedrooms, but in exchange, we get a healthcare system that actually watches over us while we dream.

When to Go to the Lab

With the explosive rise of home sleep testing, wearable tracking, and remote monitoring, it is tempting to conclude that the traditional sleep laboratory is a relic of the past. If we can diagnose sleep apnoea with a device the size of a smartphone in the comfort of our own beds, why would anyone ever choose to spend a night in a hospital, glued to electrodes, watched by a stranger? The narrative of healthcare at home is so compelling that it threatens to overshadow the reality of clinical necessity. The truth is that while the bedroom is the new front line, the laboratory remains the ultimate court of appeal. There are boundaries to what can be achieved in the home, and understanding those boundaries is a matter of life and death.

The fundamental limitation of the home sleep apnoea test (HSAT) is that it is a tool designed for a single purpose: to find Obstructive Sleep Apnoea (OSA). It is a confirmational tool. If a middle-aged man who snores loudly and falls asleep at traffic lights takes a home test, the result is almost certainly going to be positive. The pre-test probability is high, and the device is simply putting a number on the obvious. But sleep medicine is not just about snoring. It encompasses a vast spectrum of neurological and physiological disorders that a simple breathing monitor will completely miss.

The most critical blind spot of the home test is its inability to measure sleep itself. Most home devices measure airflow and oxygen, but they do not measure brain waves (EEG). They rely on the device's internal clock or the patient's own report to guess when sleep began. This creates a dangerous mathematical loophole. The severity of sleep apnoea is calculated by dividing the number of choking events by the hours of sleep. If a patient with severe insomnia spends eight hours in bed but only sleeps for two hours, the home device might assume they slept for eight. This dilutes the data, making a severe disease look mild or non-existent. For the patient who reports I sleep terribly, but the test said I'm fine, the lab is the only place to solve the mystery.

In the laboratory, the Type 1 Polysomnogram (PSG) measures sleep stage by stage. It captures the transition from wake to light sleep, the descent into deep delta sleep, and the paralysis of REM. This allows the clinician to diagnose sleep state misperception or paradoxical insomnia; a condition where the patient feels they have been awake all night, but the EEG proves they were asleep. Seeing this objective reality can be a profound therapeutic moment for the patient, breaking the cycle of anxiety about sleep loss.

Then there is the terrifying world of parasomnias. These are disorders where the brain is caught in a glitch between states. This includes sleepwalking, night terrors, and, most dangerously, REM Sleep Behaviour Disorder (RBD). In a healthy brain, a switch in the brainstem paralyses the muscles during REM sleep so that we do not act out our dreams. In patients with RBD, this switch fails. They punch, kick, scream, and leap out of bed while chasing dream enemies. This condition is not only dangerous to the patient and their bed partner, but it is also a strong early predictor of neurodegenerative diseases like Parkinson's.

A home test cannot diagnose RBD. It might see movement, but it cannot correlate that movement with the dream state. To diagnose it, you need video-polysomnography. You need a synchronised recording of the brain in REM sleep, the muscle tone on the chin and legs (EMG) showing a lack of paralysis, and the video evidence of the behaviour. You need a technician watching in real-time to ensure the patient does not injure themselves. This is a level of forensic surveillance that simply cannot be replicated in a bedroom.

Narcolepsy and hypersomnia represent another frontier where the lab is non-negotiable. These are disorders of sleep-wake stability. A patient with narcolepsy can fall into REM sleep instantly, sometimes collapsing in the middle of a conversation (cataplexy). Diagnosing this requires a gruelling protocol known as the Multiple Sleep Latency Test (MSLT). After a full night of supervised sleep in the lab to rule out other causes, the patient is asked to stay for the next day. They are given five opportunities to nap every two hours.

The test measures how quickly they fall asleep and, crucially, whether they go straight into REM sleep (the dream state). A normal tired person might fall asleep in ten minutes but will not dream. A narcoleptic might fall asleep in two minutes and be dreaming in three. This precise sleep architecture is the fingerprint of the disease. It requires a controlled environment, free from the distractions of the home, with a technician ensuring the patient stays awake between naps. You cannot take an MSLT on your sofa.

The laboratory is also the safety net for the medically complex. Patients with severe heart failure, advanced lung disease (e.g. COPD), or neuromuscular disorders like Motor Neurone Disease require a level of monitoring that goes beyond simple diagnostics. Their oxygen levels can drift dangerously low; their heart rhythms can become unstable. For these patients, the sleep study is not just a test; it is a medical procedure. The attended nature of the study means a highly trained physiologist is sitting ten metres away. If a lead falls off, they fix it. If the patient goes into a dangerous arrhythmia, they act.

We must also consider the distinction between central and obstructive sleep apnoea. In obstructive apnoea, the throat closes but the body tries to breathe; the chest heaves against the blockage. In central apnoea, the brain simply forgets to tell the body to breathe. The chest is still. The airway is open, but the drive is gone. This often happens in heart failure or as a side effect of opioid medication. Distinguishing between these two requires measuring respiratory effort, which is done with calibrated belts around the chest and abdomen. While some high-end home kits try to estimate this, the lab remains the gold standard for differentiation. Treating central apnoea with a standard CPAP machine can sometimes make it worse, a phenomenon known as treatment-emergent central sleep apnoea. The lab is where they sort the mechanics from the neurology.

So, when should you go to the lab? You go when the home test doesn't make sense. You go when the data says you are fine, but you feel terrible. You go when you do weird things in your sleep, e.g. shouting, punching, eating. You go when you have serious heart or lung conditions that make home testing risky. And you go when your job depends on it, i.e. pilots and train drivers often require the irrefutable proof of a lab study to clear them for duty.

The future of sleep medicine and clinical labs is a hybrid model. The decentralised clinic will handle the volume, the millions of straightforward cases of obstructive sleep apnoea. It will be the screening layer. But the sleep laboratory will evolve into a tertiary care hub. It will become smaller, more specialised, and more intensive.

We must resist the urge to view the home test as a replacement for the lab. It is a filter for the lab. It clears out the simple cases so that the experts can focus on the hard ones. In the end, there is no algorithm that can replace the watchful eye of a skilled technician and the controlled safety of the clinical environment. There are times when the bedroom is the best place to sleep, but there are also times when it is the worst place to measure.

6

Switches For Calm

NIETZSCHE

The Vagus Nerve Connection

There is a specific, universal sensation that is the enemy of sleep. It is the feeling of being tired but wired. Your body is exhausted, your eyes are heavy, and you have been lying in the dark for over an hour. But inside your chest, there is a hum: a frequency, a *low-flying panic attack* (to quote Radiohead). It is a subtle vibration of alertness that refuses to shut down. Your heart rate feels slightly too fast and you start panicking about it. Your thoughts are darting around like wasps in a jar.

You are physically stationary, but biologically, you are sprinting.

To understand why this sometimes happens, and how the next generation of sleep technology intends to fix it, we have to look away from the brain and down towards the neck, to a wandering cable of fibres known as the vagus nerve. The human nervous system is often described using the metaphor of a car. We have an accelerator and a brake. The accelerator is the *Sympathetic Nervous System*. This is the ancient fight or flight mechanism we are all well educated about. When this is activated, it floods the system with cortisol and adrenaline. It dilates the pupils, tenses the muscles, and speeds up the heart. It prepares the animal to survive a threat. It is designed for short, sharp bursts of intensity.

The brake is the *Parasympathetic Nervous System*, and this is something we should all know much more about. This is the rest and digest mode. When this system takes over, the heart rate slows, blood pressure drops, digestion resumes, and the body enters a state of recovery and repair. Critically, this is the only state in which sleep initiation is possible. You cannot fall asleep while you are running away from a tiger, and you cannot fall asleep if your body *thinks* it is running away from a tiger.

The vagus nerve is the physical handbrake of this system. Its name comes from the Latin for wandering, because it meanders on a long, winding path from the brainstem, down through the neck, past the vocal cords, around the heart and lungs, and deep into the abdomen. It is the longest cranial nerve in the body, a superhighway of information connecting the brain to almost every major organ. Never heard of it before? Don't worry, neither had I until recent times.

For most of human history, we believed that this system was autonomic, meaning automatic and beyond our conscious control. We thought the heart beat at the speed it wanted to, and we were just passengers. But we now know this is not true. The vagus nerve is a bidirectional channel, more of an optical fibre than a copper wire. The brain sends signals down to the organs (top-down), but the organs also send signals up to the brain (bottom-up). In fact, the scientific consensus is that eighty to ninety per cent of the fibres in the vagus nerve are afferent, meaning they carry information from the body's organs to the brain.

This is the key to the 'switch for calm'. If we can stimulate the vagus nerve, we can send a false signal to the brain that says, *We are safe. We are calm. It is time to sleep*. We could manually pull the handbrake, but the problem with modern life is that our accelerator is jammed on, pedal to the metal. We live in a world of chronic, low-grade stress: the email notification, the deadline, the blue light, the traffic jam; these are all micro-aggressions that tickle and poke the sympathetic nervous system. We spend our days bathed in a soup of stress hormones that our body can't decipher. So by the time 11pm rolls around, we have so much momentum in the fight direction that simply lying down is not enough to stop the car. We need a stronger set of brakes, and air bags.

Traditional advice for this is top-down. We are told to meditate, to count sheep, to rationalise our worries away, to keep a note pad by the side of the bed. We try to use the thinking brain (the prefrontal cortex) to talk the emotional brain (the amygdala) off the ledge. This is hard work and counterintuitive. It requires cognitive effort at a time when we are depleted. It is like trying to stop a runaway train by standing in front of it and asking it nicely to halt.

The new wave of sleep technology takes a bottom-up approach. It ignores the thoughts and targets the biology directly. It asks: where can we access this nerve, and how can we turn it on? It turns out, the vagus nerve is surprisingly accessible. While the main trunk runs deep in the neck next to the carotid artery (a dangerous place to mess around), a small branch of it, known as the auricular branch, surfaces in the ear. Specifically, it feeds the skin of the cymba concha: that little hollow just above the ear canal. This is the only place on the surface of the human body where a cranial nerve is exposed to the outside world. It is a biological USB port.

This anatomical quirk has given rise to a field called neuromodulation. By applying specific stimuli; electrical, vibrational, or even sonic, to the vagus nerve, we can force the parasympathetic system to engage. We can measure this engagement through a metric called Heart Rate Variability (HRV).

When the vagus nerve fires, it releases a neurotransmitter called acetylcholine onto the pacemaker cells of the heart.

This increases the time between heartbeats. A high HRV means your heart is responsive and flexible, dancing between the beat of the accelerator and the brake. A low HRV means your heart is locked into a rigid, metronomic rhythm driven by stress. The goal of vagus nerve technology is to boost HRV. It is to increase vagal tone. Think of vagal tone like muscle tone. A person with high vagal tone can recover from stress quickly. Something frightens them, their heart races, but five minutes later they are calm again. A person with low vagal tone gets stuck. They get an angry email at 5pm, and their heart is still pounding at 10pm.

The implications for sleep are profound. If we can artificially boost vagal tone in the hour before bed, we can drastically reduce sleep onset latency, which is the time it takes to fall asleep. We can transition the body from the red zone to the green zone mechanically. This shifts the responsibility of relaxation. Instead of trying to relax (which is a paradox, because trying is a form of tension) you simply activate the switch. You let the physiology lead, and the psychology follows. You don't calm your mind to slow your heart; you slow your heart to calm your mind.

We are seeing this logic applied in various modalities and I have tried a few of the wearables at home and at tech shows. Some are electrical, sending tiny, imperceptible currents through the skin. Some are resonant, using sound waves that vibrate in the chest cavity to stimulate the nerve fibres in the lungs. Some are breathing-based, using the fact that the vagus nerve is activated during long, slow exhalations.

The Vagus Nerve Connection is the foundation of the modern calm technology stack. It validates the idea that stress is not just in your head; it is in your nerves, your gut, and your heart rate. And because it is physical, it can be treated physically.

As we move through this chapter, we will explore the specific tools that leverage this connection. We will look at ear clips that zap you into serenity, haptic engines that purr like cats, and biofeedback screens that let you drive your own heart. But they all share the same underlying mechanism; they are all attempts to reach into the frantic machinery of the modern body and firmly, gently, pull the brake. They are the switches that turn off the world so that we can finally leave it.

Neuromodulation at Home

For decades, the idea of using electricity to alter the state of the brain was the stuff of science fiction, Hollywood horror shows, or severe psychiatry. It conjured images of heavy machinery, clinical restraints, and the brute force of electroconvulsive therapy. The notion that you could safely, gently, and effectively zap your nervous system into a state of relaxation while sitting on your sofa was unimaginable.

Yet, this is precisely the promise of the emerging field of home neuromodulation. Specifically, we are witnessing the democratisation of a technology known as transcutaneous auricular vagus nerve stimulation (taVNS). It is a mouthful of a name for a device that looks surprisingly like a standard pair of headphones, or wearables, but which acts as a digital pharmaceutical download.

The journey of Vagus Nerve Stimulation (VNS) began as an extreme set of treatments in the hospital environment. Since the late 1990s, neurosurgeons have implanted pacemaker-like devices into the chests of patients with severe, drug-resistant epilepsy. Wires were threaded up the neck and wrapped around the vagus nerve. The device would send regular pulses of electricity to the nerve, which successfully reduced seizure frequency and, interestingly, often improved the patient's mood. It was an invasive, surgical procedure reserved for the sickest patients.

The breakthrough came when researchers realised they didn't need to cut the skin to reach the nerve. Because the auricular branch of the vagus nerve surfaces in the ear, they found they could stimulate it through the skin (transcutaneously) using special electrodes clipped to the ear. This changed everything by taking a surgical implant and turning it into a wearable gadget.

So, what does this look like in the modern bedroom? The device typically consists of a small control unit, often just your smartphone connected via Bluetooth, and an earpiece. The earpiece might clip onto the tragus (the little flap of cartilage covering the ear canal) or nestle into the cymba concha (the upper hollow of the ear). The mechanism is subtle but powerful. The electrical stimulation triggers the release of inhibitory neurotransmitters, such as GABA, which act as the brain's natural sedative. Simultaneously, it dampens the production of norepinephrine, the chemical associated with alertness and anxiety. It effectively tells the brain's threat detection centre, the amygdala, to stand down.

For the person trying to sleep, the experience is often described as a parasympathetic nudge. Unlike a sleeping pill, which knocks you out with a chemical sledgehammer, taVNS does not force unconsciousness. You can use it and still drive a car or read a book. Instead, it removes the friction of anxiety. Users often report that after fifteen or twenty minutes of stimulation, they simply feel ready to go to sleep. The racing thoughts slow down, the physical tension in the shoulders evaporates, and the chest feels lighter. The consumer market for these devices is currently in a wild west phase. We are seeing a split between certified medical devices and wellness gadgets. On one side, there are companies seeking FDA clearance to treat specific conditions like migraines or Post-Traumatic Stress Disorder (PTSD). These devices are rigorous, expensive, and often require a prescription. On the other side, there is a flood of consumer-grade ear clips appearing on the market that promise to 'hack your stress' or 'boost your Zen'.

The difference lies in the waveform. The vagus nerve is picky. It responds best to specific frequencies and pulse widths. A medical-grade device delivers a precise, calibrated signal that has been proven in clinical trials to activate the nerve fibres. A cheap consumer knock-off might just be vibrating your skin without actually engaging the nervous system. As with all early-stage tech, the buyer must be wary. The protocol for sleep usually involves a twenty to thirty-minute session right before bed. You might clip the device on while you brush your teeth and get into pyjamas. You sit in bed, perhaps reading or meditating, while the device hums away on your ear. The physical sensation of the tingling becomes a cue for the brain: *this is the feeling of winding down.* It potentially then becomes a Pavlovian response.

We are also seeing the emergence of closed-loop taVNS. This connects the stimulation to the biofeedback we discussed in earlier chapters. Imagine an earbud that measures your heart rate variability in real-time. If it detects that your HRV is low and you are stressed, it automatically initiates a gentle stimulation session to bring you back to baseline. It stops when your biometrics show you are calm. This removes the guesswork. The device manages your arousal levels autonomously.

There are limitations. The dose of electricity required varies wildly from person to person. Some people are super-responders who feel a profound wave of relaxation within minutes. Others feel nothing but an itchy ear. The anatomy of the ear also varies; if the electrode doesn't make perfect contact with the specific nerve branch, the effect is lost. It is not a magic wand that works for everyone, every time.

Looking forward, the form factor is destined to disappear. The major tech giants are all filing patents for headphones and earbuds with integrated biometric sensors and health features and I saw a few of these at CES this year (2026). It is inevitable that future generations of standard consumer earbuds; i.e. the ones you already use to listen to music will include taVNS capabilities.

Imagine listening to a sleep story or a podcast on your earbuds, and beneath the audio, a silent, sub-perceptual electrical signal is gently coaxing your vagus nerve into relaxation. The hardware is already in your ears; it just needs to be taught how to speak the language of the nervous system.

Neuromodulation at home represents a profound shift in how we manage our own biology. It treats electricity as a therapy and it acknowledges that we are bio-electrical beings. Sometimes, the best way to fix a software problem (anxiety) is to tweak the hardware (the nerve). For the insomniac staring at the ceiling, waiting for the chemical crash of a pill, the ability to simply press a button and dial down the noise of the world is a potentially powerful liberation.

Biofeedback Loops

The fundamental problem with stress is that it is often invisible to the person suffering from it. We are notoriously bad at judging our own physiological state. You might be sitting on the sofa watching television, convinced you are relaxing, while your heart is hammering away at eighty beats per minute and your blood pressure is simmering near the red line. We have lost the ability to feel the difference between stopped and idling.

This disconnect between our perception and our biology creates a dangerous blind spot when we try to sleep. We lie in bed thinking, *I am calm, why can't I sleep?* The answer is that while your mind might be quiet, your nervous system is shouting about something that happened hours ago. This is where biofeedback comes in. It acts as a mirror for your autonomic nervous system, making the invisible visible.

The dashboard for this new technology is a metric we have already touched on: Heart Rate Variability (HRV). To recap, HRV is the variation in time between consecutive heartbeats. Unlike a metronome, a healthy heart is an irregular heart. It speeds up slightly when you inhale and slows down when you exhale. This dance is called Respiratory Sinus Arrhythmia. It is a sign that your parasympathetic nervous system (the brake) is engaging with your sympathetic nervous system (the accelerator). A high HRV means you are flexible, adaptive, and recovering. A low HRV means you are rigid, stressed, and potentially stuck in survival mode.

Biofeedback takes this complex data stream and turns it into a simple game. You clip a sensor to your ear or strap a monitor to your chest, and you look at a screen. The screen might show a garden. When your HRV is low (stress), the garden is withered and grey. When your HRV is high (calm), the flowers bloom and the colours become vibrant. Or it might be a simple line graph that you have to keep above a certain threshold.

The loop works like this: The sensor reads your heart. The screen shows you the state of your heart. You see that you are stressed. You change your behaviour, usually by changing your breathing, to influence the signal. You see the screen change instantly. This visual confirmation reinforces the behaviour.

The most effective lever in this loop is breathing. The heart and the lungs are mechanically and neurologically coupled. When you take a slow, deep breath, you increase the pressure in your chest and stimulate the vagus nerve, which tells the heart to slow down. By timing your breathing to a specific rhythm, you can synchronise your heart rate with your breath cycle. This state is called coherence or resonance.

For most adults, this resonance frequency occurs at roughly six breaths per minute; specifically, a five-second inhale and a five-second exhale (a bit like military style box-breathing techniques). When you breathe at this rate, your HRV swells to its maximum amplitude. The line on the biofeedback screen turns into a perfect, smooth sine wave. You are literally tuning your nervous system like an instrument. The technology that facilitates this has moved from the clinic to the pocket. In the past, biofeedback required a desktop computer and a mess of wires in a therapist's office. Now, it is an app on your phone paired with a Bluetooth sensor. There are devices that act as pacers, guiding your breath with expanding and contracting shapes or rising and falling tones.

The power of the biofeedback loop is that it bypasses the intellect therefore you do not need to try to relax; you just play the game. You focus on making the flower bloom or keeping the green light on. In doing so, you are forcing your biology into a parasympathetic state. It is a back door into meditation for people who hate meditation. If you cannot sit still and watch your thoughts, you can almost certainly sit still and watch your score.

The goal of this training is not to become dependent on the device, but to train the 'muscle' of the vagus nerve. Just as lifting weights makes a bicep stronger, spending twenty minutes a day in a state of high coherence trains your nervous system to access that state more easily. This is the concept of neuroplasticity applied to the heart. Over time, the body learns what calm feels like, even if you can't remember. Eventually, you take the training wheels off. You find yourself in a stressful meeting or lying in bed unable to sleep, and you simply shift your breathing into that six-breath-per-minute rhythm. You don't need the screen to tell you it's working because you can feel the shift.

This technology creates a virtuous circle. You use the device to calm down before bed, which lowers your sleep onset latency. You sleep better, which improves your baseline HRV the next morning. A higher baseline HRV makes you more resilient to stress the next day, which makes it easier to wind down the next night. You are spinning the flywheel of sleep improvement in the right direction.

In the programmable sanctuary of the next decade, biofeedback will likely be integrated into the environment. Your smart lights might pulse slowly at six times per minute to guide your breathing as you read. Your mattress might gently inflate and deflate to pace your rhythm. But until then, the simple act of watching your own heart on a screen and learning to slow it down remains one of the most potent skills a modern human can master. It proves that 'peace' is not just a concept; it is a quantitative metric, and it is one you can improve with technology.

Haptics and Touch

Touch is the first sense to develop in the womb. Long before a foetus can see or hear it can feel, it is our most primitive and fundamental language of safety. When a baby cries, we do not show it a spreadsheet explaining why it is safe, nor do we play it a podcast about emotional regulation. We pick it up gently and we rock it calmly. We hold it close to our chest, heartbeat to heartbeat. The physical sensation of being held, of rhythmic movement and warmth, sends a signal to the brainstem that bypasses logic entirely. It says: *You are not alone. You are safe.*

In the modern world, however, we are increasingly touch-starved. We spend our days interacting with glass screens and plastic keyboards. We live in a visual and auditory dominance, bombarded by pixels and soundwaves, but physically isolated. When we go to bed, we lie there alone, or next to a partner we might not touch all night, and expect our nervous systems to settle down without the tactile reassurance they evolved to expect.

This is where the field of haptics enters the sleep equation. Haptics is the science of communicating through touch. For most of the last decade, haptic technology was used primarily to annoy us. It was the sharp, jagged buzz of a phone notification in a pocket, or the phantom tap on a wrist telling us to stand up. It was designed to alert, to startle, and to demand attention. Cortisol trigger 101.

The new wave of sleep technology is flipping this script. It is exploring affective haptics; vibrations and pressures designed not to alert, but to soothe. It is the digital manifestation of the hug. The biological mechanism here is Deep Pressure Stimulation (DPS) and rhythmic entrainment. We see the low-tech version of this in the weighted blanket. These heavy quilts, filled with glass beads or plastic pellets, weigh anywhere from five to ten kilograms. When you lie under one, the weight provides a uniform, firm pressure across the entire body.

To the nervous system, this feels like a continuous, firm embrace. It stimulates proprioceptors; the sensors that tell your brain where your body is in space. This flood of proprioceptive data has a grounding effect. It increases the production of serotonin (the precursor to melatonin) and decreases cortisol. It physically forces the body to be still, reducing the restlessness and thrashing that often accompany insomnia.

But blankets are passive. The high-tech frontier is active haptics. These are wearable devices (wristbands, chest straps, or even small pebbles you hold in your hand) that emit low-frequency vibrations. Unlike the jarring buzz of a text message, these vibrations are slow, rolling, and rhythmic. They mimic the frequency of a resting heart rate or the purr of a cat. The concept is similar to music, but for your skin. Just as listening to a slow song can slow your heart rate through entrainment, feeling a slow rhythm on your wrist can encourage your nervous system to sync up with the beat. The device acts as a metronome for your mood.

One of the leading theories is that these vibrations target the insular cortex, the part of the brain responsible for interoception (the sense of the internal state of the body). By providing a steady, safe external rhythm, the device interrupts the feedback loop of anxiety. The brain focuses on the sensation of the vibration rather than the sensation of the racing heart. It is a distraction therapy that operates below the level of conscious thought.

The most dramatic application of haptic technology is in the treatment of nightmares, particularly for those suffering from PTSD. For a veteran or a trauma survivor, sleep is not a refuge; it is a battlefield. Nightmares can re-traumatise the brain every night, spiking the heart rate to 180 beats per minute and drenching the sleeper in sweat. They wake up terrified, exhausted, and afraid to go back to sleep. Enter NightWare; this is a prescription digital therapeutic in the USA that runs on an Apple Watch. It uses the watch's heart rate and movement sensors to build a profile of the user's sleep. It learns to recognise the specific physiological signature of a nightmare.

When the algorithm detects that a nightmare is beginning; the heart rate spikes and the movement becomes erratic, it intervenes. But it does not wake the patient up with a loud alarm, which would be cruel. Instead, it delivers a gentle, specific haptic pulse to the wrist. It is just enough sensation to arouse the brain out of the deep dreaming state, breaking the narrative of the nightmare, but not enough to fully wake the patient up. The sleeper might shift position, sigh, and fall back into a safe, dreamless sleep, never knowing the intervention happened. In the morning, they simply know they rested. This is haptics acting as a sentry. It is a digital hand on the shoulder that says, *It's okay, it's just a dream.*

We are also seeing haptics integrated into the bed itself. 'Smart' mattresses now come with arrays of vibration motors embedded in the foam. These can act as a silent alarm clock, gently buzzing you awake without disturbing your partner. But more importantly, they can be used for vibro-acoustic relaxation. Before bed, the mattress can gently shudder and hum at specific frequencies designed to relax the large muscle groups of the back and legs. It creates a physical sensation of dissolving tension. Some systems link this to the user's breathing rate, creating a biofeedback loop where the bed physically guides you into a slower rhythm. You are literally being rocked to sleep by a robot bed. Nothing to be concerned about there, then.

The power of haptics lies in its immediacy. You can ignore a sound. You can close your eyes to a light. But it is very hard to ignore a physical sensation. It cuts through the cognitive noise. When a device vibrates slowly against your sternum or your wrist, it commands the attention of the nervous system in a way that is ancient and undeniable.

As we move forward, we will likely see haptic clothing such as pyjamas with integrated actuators that can deliver a massage or a reassuring squeeze on command. We are moving from a world of hard, dead surfaces to a world of responsive, tactile environments. For the anxious sleeper, this offers a new kind of medicine. It is not a pill you swallow, but a feeling you wear.

Modern Meditation Tech

We are living through a strange historical irony: The very device that destroyed our attention spans aka the smartphone, is now the primary tool we are using to try and get them back. We doom-scroll through anxiety-inducing news feeds for an hour, have a notification pop up with a loud ping every few minutes, and then, with a tap of a finger, we open an app that promises to undo all the cognitive damage with just ten minutes of blue-skied serenity. This is the paradox of modern meditation technology. It is an attempt to use the cause of the problem as the solution. However, for the millions of people who find the concept of sitting in silence either boring or terrifying, this digital intervention is a necessary bridge.

The landscape of digital mindfulness is divided into two distinct categories: the software that guides you, and the hardware that measures you.

On the software side, the giants of the industry such as Headspace and Calm have fundamentally rebranded meditation (noting that I am writing this book whilst listening to focus music on Headspace). They have taken a practice that was once associated with incense, robes, and esoteric spirituality, and repackaged it as gym for the mind. For the sleep-deprived, the most significant innovation from these apps is not actually meditation, but the Sleep Story. This is a modern reinvention of the bedtime story, but with a specific engineering purpose. It uses a technique known as cognitive shuffling or narrative transportation.

When you cannot sleep, your brain is usually stuck in a loop of hot cognition, i.e. worrying about the future, replaying the past, or obsessing over the fact that you are not sleeping. A sleep story breaks this loop by giving the brain a neutral narrative to follow. It might be a story about a train journey across Siberia, or a description of a lavender field in Provence, read by a celebrity with a soothing voice (noting they haven't hired me yet and I think I could be quite good at this). The plot is deliberately boring where nothing exciting happens. There is no conflict, no climax, and no resolution; it is narrative sedative. It occupies the brain just enough to stop the worrying, but not enough to keep it awake. It is a digital lullaby that outsources the heavy lifting of quieting the mind.

On the hardware side, the technology gets more aggressive. This is the domain of consumer EEG headbands, such as the Muse. These devices attempt to solve the single biggest problem with traditional meditation: the doubt. When a beginner tries to meditate, they sit there with their eyes closed, thinking, *Am I doing it right? Is this it? I'm just thinking about lunch, my ex, and that Alanis Morisette lyric. I'm definitely doing it wrong.* And because they cannot see their own brain, they have no feedback loop, so they often get frustrated and quit.

Neurofeedback headbands solve this by making the invisible visible. They measure the electrical activity of the brain in real-time and convert it into sound. When your brain is active and noisy (beta waves), you hear the sound of a storm; wind rushing, rain falling. When you successfully focus your attention and quiet your mind (alpha and theta waves), the storm subsides, and you hear gentle birds chirping. This creates a powerful operant conditioning loop. You are not just sitting there hoping for peace; you are playing the game of peace. When you hear the birds, your brain gets a dopamine hit of validation. *Yes, that is the state.* You learn what calm actually feels like neurologically. For the analytical, data-driven sleeper who hates ambiguity, this is a revelation. It turns relaxation into an engineering challenge that can be won.

However, there is a potential trap here. The gamification of silence can ultimately defeat the purpose of silence. If you are meditating to get a high score or to keep a streak alive on your app, you are still in a mode of striving, and you are still performing. True rest requires the cessation of effort, not just a different kind of effort. There is a risk that we become dependent on the external validation of the device, unable to self-soothe without a battery-powered headband telling us we are doing a good job.

Furthermore, there is the issue of state versus trait. These tools are excellent at creating a temporary *state* of calm, i.e. they can help you lower your cortisol right now so you can fall asleep. But the deeper promise of meditation is a lifestyle change, a permanent shift in how you relate to stress and the world. It is unclear whether playing a biofeedback game for ten minutes a day leads to that deeper transformation, or if it is simply a digital aspirin.

Ultimately, consider the role of modern meditation tech to be a set of training wheels. It is there to teach you the feeling of the brake pedal. It helps you carve the neural pathway of relaxation through the jungle of modern distraction. The goal should not be to use the app forever, but to use it until you no longer need it. My problem is always the opposite one, I find it really hard to build good habits and actually use these technologies daily without fail.

In the programmable sanctuary, these tools have a place on the nightstand. They are the emergency switches we can flip when the internal noise gets too loud. They remind us that the mind is not a fixed entity, but a mechanism that can be tuned, quieted, and steered towards the darkness of sleep. They prove that while technology may have broken our sleep, it is also, in its own beeping, chirping way, trying to help us fix it.

7

Engineering Dreams

> We are moving from the age of interpreting dreams to the age of engineering them.

ADAM HAAR HOROWITZ, MIT MEDIA LAB

The Science of Dream Influence

For centuries, dreams were viewed as messages from the gods, or later, as the bubbling up of the subconscious mind, a chaotic theatre where our deepest fears and desires played out in symbolic form. Freud called them the 'road to the unconscious'. But for the modern neuroscientist, dreams are something far more functional and far less mystical. They are the sound of the brain saving its work.

We used to think of sleep as a passive state, a period where the brain simply shut down to save energy, like a car parked in a garage. We now know this is dangerously incorrect. The sleeping brain is a hive of frenetic activity. It is during sleep that the fragile, temporary memories formed during the day are transferred from the short-term storage of the hippocampus to the long-term hard drive of the neocortex. This process is called systems consolidation: It is the difference between remembering a phone number for five minutes and remembering it for fifty years.

Until recently, we believed this process was a black box; something that happened automatically behind closed doors, inaccessible to the outside world. But a revolutionary technique known as Targeted Memory Reactivation (TMR) has pried the door open. It has proven that we can not only watch this process happen, but we can also reach in and steer it.

The foundational experiment that established this field sounds like a parlour trick.

Researchers had participants play a memory game, learning the locations of card pairs on a computer screen. As they learned the cards, the room was flooded with the scent of roses. That night, the participants slept in the lab. While they were in Deep Slow Wave Sleep (the stage most critical for memory), the researchers puffed the same rose scent into their noses. The results were undeniable. The next morning, the participants who received the scent cue during sleep remembered the card locations significantly better than those who did not. The smell acted as a specific key, unlocking the specific memory trace in the hippocampus and forcing the brain to replay that memory over and over again during the night. The scent didn't teach them anything new; it simply told the brain, 'Save this file, not that one'.

While smell is a powerful trigger because of its direct link to the brain's emotional centre, it is impractical for the average bedroom. You cannot easily program a smell. Sound, however, is infinitely programmable. Subsequent studies have replicated the effect using auditory cues. Imagine learning to play a melody on the piano. Every time you hit a correct key, a specific tone plays. That night, while you sleep, a device plays that same melody quietly; too quietly to wake you, but loud enough for the auditory cortex to hear. The brain hears the tune, recognizes the pattern, and reactivates the motor neurons associated with the finger movements. You wake up playing the song better than when you went to bed.

This is the core of TMR, it relies on the brain's susceptibility to external input during Non-Rapid Eye Movement (NREM) sleep. During this phase, the brain is generating slow oscillations; massive, synchronised waves of electrical activity. Riding on top of these slow waves are faster bursts called spindles. It is the precise coupling of the slow wave and the spindle that drives the memory transfer. TMR works by triggering this coupling at the exact moment the relevant memory is cued.

The implications for the programmable sanctuary of the bedroom are staggering. We are moving from an era where we engineered the room to help us sleep, to an era where we engineer the room to help us learn. The bedroom becomes a classroom. A student studying Spanish vocabulary could have the specific words they struggled with pulsed into their ears during the deep delta waves of the night. A stroke victim relearning how to walk could have the neural pathways for movement reinforced while they rest.

However, there is a biological cost. The brain has a limited bandwidth for consolidation. We cannot save everything. Sleep is as much about forgetting; pruning away the useless trivia of the day, as it is about remembering. If we artificially boost the memory of a card game or a piano tune, are we displacing something else? Are we overwriting the subtle emotional processing that usually happens during that time?

TMR suggests that sleep is not a monolith: It is a programmable interface. We can tag specific memories for priority processing. This dissolves the boundary between the waking self and the sleeping self. The self that wants to learn French during the day can recruit the self that sleeps at night to finish the job. Sounds like it was derived from the TV show *Severance*.

Currently, this technology is moving from the academic lab to the consumer headset. Devices are entering the market that track your sleep stages in real-time and deliver pink noise pulses or specific audio cues at the precise millisecond of the slow-wave peak. They claim to boost memory retention by twenty or thirty per cent. But the real revolution is the shift in perspective. We are ceasing to view dreams and sleep patterns as random static. We are seeing them as a data stream, and like any data stream, if you know the code, you can edit it. TMR is the first reliable cursor we have for the editing of the sleeping mind. It proves that the learning process does not have to end when we close our eyes. In fact, if we engineer the soundscape correctly, the real work might just be getting started.

As we explore the next sections in this chapter, we will see how this capability expands from simple memory reinforcement to the rewriting of emotional trauma and the deliberate incubation of creativity.

Therapy for Nightmares

For most of us, a nightmare is a momentary glitch, just a frightening sequence of images that wakes us up, heart pounding, only to fade within minutes as reality reasserts itself. But for millions of people, particularly those suffering from PTSD, nightmares are not glitches, they are insidious. They are a nightly re-enactment of the worst moment of their lives, a broken record that skips and repeats the same horrific loop with high-fidelity sensory precision. The prevalence of this suffering is staggering. It affects combat veterans, survivors of assault, and victims of accidents. The impact goes beyond the terror of the dream itself. The fear of the nightmare creates a fear of sleep. Patients develop somniphobia, consciously or unconsciously sabotaging their own rest to avoid the theatre of the trauma. This sleep deprivation then worsens the PTSD symptoms during the day, creating a vicious cycle of anxiety and exhaustion that is notoriously difficult to treat with medication.

The gold standard treatment for this condition is a psychological intervention known as Imagery Rehearsal Therapy (IRT). It is elegant in its simplicity; the patient sits with a therapist while awake and writes down the narrative of their recurring nightmare in detail. Then, they rewrite the ending. If the nightmare involves being chased down a dark alley by an attacker, the patient might rewrite the script so that the attacker turns into a harmless puppy, or the dreamer suddenly gains the ability to fly and soars away to safety. The patient then spends time every day visualising this new, safe version of the dream. The goal is to use neuroplasticity to overwrite the traumatic memory trace with a new, neutral or positive one. When the brain starts to play the nightmare at night, it theoretically switches tracks to the new ending.

IRT is effective, but it is not perfect, and it is time consuming and expensive. It relies on the patient's ability to vividly imagine the new scenario and, crucially, on the sleeping brain's ability to remember that new scenario in the midst of REM sleep emotional arousal. Roughly thirty per cent of patients do not respond at all to IRT in its current form. The trauma is too loud; the new script is too quiet. This is where technology is stepping in to bridge the gap. We are seeing the marriage of IRT with TMR. The logic is straightforward: if we can use a sound cue to help someone remember a card game (as discussed in the previous section), why can't we use a sound cue to help them remember the new ending to their nightmare?

A landmark study published in 2022 demonstrated exactly this. Researchers in Switzerland worked with patients suffering from chronic nightmares. All patients underwent the standard IRT. However, half of the group added a technological layer. While they practised their new, positive dream endings during the day, this group listened to a specific sound; a neutral piano chord played every ten seconds. This created a strong associative link: *Piano chord = Safety or Piano chord = Flying away.*

Then came the intervention. The patients wore a wireless headband to sleep that monitored their brainwaves. When the algorithm detected that the patient had entered REM sleep (the stage where nightmares occur), it began to play that same piano chord quietly through bone-conduction headphones. It played the sound every ten seconds, just loud enough for the brain to register, but not loud enough to wake the dreamer.

The results were transformative. The group that received the sound cues during sleep had significantly fewer nightmares than the group that only did the therapy. More importantly, they reported more positive dreams. The sound acted as a lifeline thrown into the dream. It triggered the specific memory of the safe ending right at the moment the brain was deciding which script to run. It tipped the balance from trauma to triumph.

These days you may hear of the development of consumer-facing nightmare therapeutics. These are not just headbands; they are integrated software platforms. A patient might use a Virtual Reality (VR) headset during the day to visually build their new dream scenario, immersing themselves in a 3D world where they are safe and powerful. The VR experience is paired with a specific audio track. At night, a lightweight sleep mask plays that track during REM. The use of VR is particularly potent because it engages the visual cortex far more intensely than simple imagination. For a trauma survivor who has frozen their imagination as a defence mechanism, VR provides the visual scaffolding they need to build a new reality.

This technology also allows for closed-loop intervention. The device doesn't just play the sound blindly. It monitors the heart rate and movement. If it detects the physiological rising panic of a nightmare beginning, it can dynamically trigger the safety cue. It is a responsive system, intervening only when the emotional temperature of the dream gets too high. The implications extend beyond clinical PTSD. We all experience stress dreams or anxiety dreams such as the classic teeth falling out or unprepared for an exam scenarios. These are minor failures of emotional processing. Future dream hygiene devices could allow us to program safety cues that gently steer our dreams away from anxiety and towards confidence or resolution. Gosh, I could have used these during my PhD years.

However, the therapy for nightmares highlights a critical nuance in dream engineering. We are not inceptioning a totally new idea into the brain, like the movie. We are helping the brain select between options it already has. The patient has to do the work of creating the new script first. The technology is simply the delivery mechanism that ensures the new script arrives on stage at the right time. It transforms the bedroom from a place of passive suffering into a laboratory of healing. For the nightmare sufferer, the night has always been the enemy. This technology offers a truce, as it suggests that with the right programming, the sleeping brain can heal the wounds that the waking mind cannot reach. The piano chord in the dark is not just a sound; it is a signal that the story can be changed.

Targeted Dream Incubation

If you study the biographies of the great innovators of history like the surrealist painters, the quantum physicists, the inventors of the light bulb, you find a recurring, peculiar habit. They all seemed to be obsessed with the edge of sleep.

Thomas Edison, a man famous for claiming that sleep was a waste of time, utilised a technique to mine his own subconscious. He would sit in an armchair with a heavy steel ball in his hand. As he drifted off, his muscle tone would relax, the ball would crash to the floor, and the noise would wake him up. He would immediately grab a notebook and write down the strange, hallucinatory thoughts that were swirling in his mind at that precise moment. Salvador Dalí used a heavy key and a metal plate to achieve the same effect. They were both fishing in the waters of hypnagogia.

Hypnagogia, or the N1 stage of sleep, is the twilight zone between being awake and being asleep. It is a fleeting state, usually lasting only a few minutes and to the casual observer, it looks like dozing off (or checking your eyelids). But neurologically, it is a unique state of consciousness characterised by phenomenological unpredictability. The rigid, logical barriers of the waking prefrontal cortex dissolve and the brain becomes hyper-associative. Concepts that are normally kept in separate filing cabinets like gravity and violins suddenly slide together. This is the engine room of creativity.

For a century, the Edison method was the only way to access this state: a crude mechanical interrupt. You could catch the dream, but you couldn't control it. Today, we have moved from fishing to farming. We have entered the era of Targeted Dream Incubation (TDI).

The breakthrough came from the MIT Media Lab with a device called Dormio. It looks like a sci-fi glove, wrapped with sensors that track muscle tone, heart rate, and skin conductance. These sensors act as a precise altimeter for the descent into sleep. They can detect the exact moment a person slips from wakefulness into the N1 hypnagogic state. But unlike Edison's steel ball, Dormio does not just wake you up. It talks to you. The protocol works like this: You lie down, wearing the glove, and a nearby robot or app speaks a prompt, e.g. 'Remember to think of a tree'. You drift off and the sensors watch your physiology change. As you enter the dream state, the device waits for a few minutes to let the dream imagery generate, and then it wakes you up, but not fully, just enough to pull you back to the surface. It asks you to record what you were thinking, then it lets you drift back down again, whispering the prompt once more: 'Remember to think of a tree'.

This creates a semi-lucid loop, you are hovering on the threshold of consciousness, dipping in and out of the dream state, with the machine repeatedly injecting a specific seed idea into the soil of your mind. The results of the initial experiments were startling. When prompted to think of a tree, participants did not just see a static image of an oak. The hypnagogic brain took the prompt and ran with it. One participant reported dreaming of 'trees made of glass shattering'. Another saw 'a tree that was also a giant hand'. Another became the tree, feeling their roots growing into the earth.

Crucially, when these participants were tested on creative tasks after the nap, such as 'list as many creative uses for a brick as you can', they significantly outperformed those who had just stayed awake or those who had napped without the prompt. The incubation effect had primed their brains for divergent thinking.

This validates a theory that dream researchers have held for decades: the sleeping brain is not just replaying the past; it is simulating possible futures. We are a probability engine that runs *what if* scenarios without the constraints of physics or social logic. By using TDI, we are essentially feeding a search query into this biological supercomputer.

The implications for the 'programmable sanctuary' are profound. We are looking at a future where the bedroom doubles as a creative studio. An architect stuck on a design problem could program their room to incubate solutions involving structural tension or light. A writer suffering from writer's block could seed their sleep with the theme of their novel. This is a fundamental shift in our relationship with sleep. For the entirety of human history, sleep has been viewed as offline time; it was a time of absence from the rest of the community. TDI reframes sleep as a different kind of online; a processing state that is active, accessible, and steerable, and I daresay also manipulatable.

This technology forces us to confront the mechanics of subconscious influence. In the MIT study, the researchers were essentially inceptioning ideas into the subjects' minds. The participants dreamed about trees because the machine told them to. This raises the question of autonomy. If a machine can guide your dreams towards creativity, could it also guide them towards a product? Imagine a future where a smart speaker, knowing you are in the N1 state, whispers a subtle advertisement for a soft drink or a brand of sneakers, or a political leader. Because the critical faculties of the brain are offline in hypnagogia, the defence mechanisms against persuasion are lowered. The seed is planted deep. This is the dark side of dream incubation; the potential for the colonisation of the subconscious by commercial or political interests.

But for the individual user, the Dormio concept represents the ultimate tool for cognitive expansion. It democratises the genius of Dalí. You do not need to be a surrealist master to access the surrealism of your own mind; you just need the right sensor. We are seeing this technology evolve rapidly from the clunky glove of the prototype to streamlined wearables. Smartwatches and headbands are beginning to integrate hypnagogic tracking modes. They use haptic vibrations instead of steel balls to keep the user in the Goldilocks zone; deep enough to dream, but shallow enough to remember.

This fits perfectly into the integrated audit of the bedroom we discussed in Chapter 4. The lighting, the sound, and now the sensors are all aligned to support a specific mental state. The room becomes a vessel for liminal drift.

Targeted Dream Incubation suggests that we have vastly underestimated the utility of the transition into sleep. We rush through it, treating it as a waiting room for the main event of deep sleep. But TDI shows us that this borderland is rich with resources. It is a place where the brain is uniquely flexible, open to suggestion, and capable of forging connections that the waking mind would dismiss as impossible. By engineering this state, we are not just getting better sleep; we are getting better waking. We are retrieving the gems that usually dissolve in the morning light.

Lucid Dreaming Technology

If Targeted Memory Reactivation is about subtly editing the save file of the sleeping brain, and Targeted Dream Incubation is about whispering a suggestion to the subconscious, then

Lucid Dreaming (LD) is the ultimate act of user revolt. It is the moment the player realises they are in a game and takes control of the console.

A lucid dream is defined as a dream state in which the dreamer is fully aware that they are dreaming. In this state, the vivid, immersive sensory hallucinations of REM sleep continue, but the dreamer's critical faculties such as their logic, memory, and volition all come back online. They can fly on command, summon specific people, walk through walls, or sit down and meditate in a landscape of their own creation. It is the original, high-fidelity Virtual Reality, generated entirely by the biological hardware of the brain, with zero latency and infinite resolution.

For decades, this state was considered a rarity, a spontaneous anomaly reported by mystics or the lucky few. But as we have mapped the sleeping brain, we have discovered the neural signature of lucidity. In a normal dream, the dorsolateral prefrontal cortex (the centre of logic and self-awareness) is deactivated. This is why we accept the bizarre logic of dreams; we do not question why we are taking an exam in our pyjamas. In a lucid dream, this region lights up and the brain enters a unique hybrid state, i.e. simultaneously deep in REM at the back of the brain (visuals/emotions) and awake at the front (logic).

The promise of Lucid Dreaming Technology is to induce this hybrid state on demand. It is the quest for a lucid dream at the push of a button. And for the last ten years, the consumer sleep market has been flooded with devices claiming to provide exactly that. The reality, however, is a landscape littered with broken promises, flashing lights, and a lot of very confused sleepers. The most common form of this technology is the flashing mask. These devices operate on a simple premise: external cueing. You wear a sleep mask embedded with red LEDs. The device attempts to guess when you are in REM sleep (usually using a simple timer or movement sensor). When it thinks you are dreaming, it flashes the lights against your closed eyelids.

The theory is that the red flashing will bleed into your dream imagery. You might be dreaming of walking down a street, and suddenly the sky turns red, or a flashing police light appears. You have trained yourself during the day to recognise this signal: *Red lights mean I am dreaming.* Ideally, you see the cue, realise your state, and become lucid. In practice, these devices often fail for two reasons. First, without EEG (brainwave) sensors, they are guessing when you are in REM sleep. If they flash the lights while you are in deep sleep, you just wake up annoyed. Second, the dreaming brain is a master of rationalisation. It creates a narrative to explain the stimulus. You don't think, 'Ah, a signal from the waking world'. You think 'Look at those fireworks'. The signal is incorporated into the illusion rather than shattering it.

The failure of the light-only approach has pushed the industry towards more diverse interventions: electrical stimulation again (and not the vagus nerve this time). This is based on a landmark finding that specific brainwave frequencies (specifically Gamma waves at 40 Hz) are associated with self-awareness. In 2014, researchers found that by applying a gentle alternating current (tACS) at 40 Hz to the foreheads of sleeping volunteers, they could force the brain into a lucid state. They essentially jump-started the prefrontal cortex with a battery. This sparked a wave of DIY neurostimulation enthusiasm. Brave bio-hackers began strapping electrodes to their heads, hoping to zap themselves into god-like control of their dreams. But the transition from a controlled lab with medical-grade equipment to a bedroom device soldered in your dad's man shed is fraught with difficulty. The connection between the electrode and the skin must be perfect. The timing must be millisecond-precise. If the current is too high, it wakes the sleeper up. If it is too low, it does nothing. The lucid dream on demand remains elusive because the biological variability between humans is so vast. The current state of the art lies in closed-loop acoustic induction. This is a more sophisticated version of the flashing mask logic. Instead of lights, it uses sound. And instead of guessing, it uses real EEG sensors (like the headbands discussed in previous chapters) to confirm REM sleep.

The protocol involves a reality check training regimen. During the day, every time your phone makes a specific ping sound, you ask yourself: 'Am I dreaming?' You look at your hands, check the time, or try to float. You condition your brain to associate that specific ping with a critical state check. At night, the headband monitors your sleep architecture. It waits until you are deep in a stable REM cycle; usually in the early morning hours when dreams are longest. Then, it plays the 'ping' sound softly. You hear the ping in the dream, your conditioned reflex kicks in (Am I dreaming?), and *click*; you become lucid. Sounds easy.

But even with the best hardware, the technology is only a compass, not a pilot. It points you towards the state, but you have to step through the door. The most effective use of these devices is not as a magic pill, but as an amplifier for mental discipline. The cyborg approach created by combining a disciplined meditation practice (like the Wake Back to Bed method) with a high-precision EEG trigger, yields the highest success rates.

Why go to all this trouble? It sounds like the start of a 1980s sci-fi horror movie. Why engineer a room to let you control a hallucination? Because the applications of lucidity extend far beyond entertainment. It is the ultimate simulator. Athletes use it to practice motor skills; a skier can ski a course a hundred times in a lucid dream, firing the actual neural pathways for movement without the risk of injury. Artists use it to sculpt impossible structures. Therapists use it to help patients confront trauma safely, i.e. if you know you are dreaming, you can turn and face the monster, asking it what it represents, rather than running away.

In the context of the programmable sanctuary, lucid dreaming technology represents the final frontier of autonomy. It turns the bed into a Star Trek holodeck. It challenges the very definition of rest. If you spend eight hours flying through a city you built with your mind, have you rested? Physiologically, yes, your body was paralysed, your muscles repaired. But psychologically, you were active.

There is a philosophical tension here as well. Sleep has historically been a time of surrender, a time of letting go of the ego and the will. Lucid dreaming is the assertion of the ego into the one space where it usually dissolves. There is a risk that by colonising our sleep with our waking desires for control and productivity, we lose the chaotic, nonsensical wisdom that normal dreams provide.

However, for the dream engineer, the choice is the point. The technology does not force you to be lucid every night. It simply gives you the option. It offers a switch on the wall of the mind that says 'Manual Override'. And for the sleeper who wants to explore the furthest reaches of their own consciousness, having that switch is the ultimate luxury.

The Ethics of Dream Engineering

For the entirety of human existence, the dreamscape has been the one truly private sanctuary. It was the only place where we were completely alone, free from the gaze of the state, the pressures of the market, and the judgment of our peers. We could be locked in a prison cell, but in our sleep, we could walk on a beach. We could be penniless, but in our dreams, we could be billionaires. The skull was the final fortress of solitude, and the dream was the last unmapped wilderness. The technologies we have discussed in this chapter Targeted

Memory Reactivation, Dream Incubation, and Lucid Dreaming induction, have effectively breached that fortress. By turning the dream into a programmable interface, we have opened the door to a host of ethical dilemmas that were previously the domain of dystopian fiction. We are now forced to ask: if a dream can be engineered, who owns the engineering?

The most immediate danger is the commercialisation of the unconscious. We live in an attention economy where every waking second is commodified. Our screens, our streets, and our podcasts are saturated with advertising. The only time a corporation cannot reach us is when we are asleep. Roughly one-third of our lives is currently dead capital to the advertising industry. Dream engineering offers them a way to unlock it.

This is not a theoretical concern as we have already seen proof of concept stunts where major beverage and fast-food brands have offered free products to volunteers in exchange for them using dream incubation protocols. They provide the soundscapes and the prompts, 'dream of a refreshing mountain stream' or 'think of a flame-grilled burger' to be played during the hypnagogic state. In the waking world, we have epistemic vigilance, a critical filter that allows us to recognise an ad as an ad. We can roll our eyes, mute the volume, or intellectually reject the message. But in the N1 hypnagogic state and in REM sleep, the critical prefrontal cortex is offline. The brain is hyper-associative and suggestible so it accepts input without judgment.

If an advertisement is seeded into a dream, it bypasses the critical filter entirely. It plants the desire for a product deep in the emotional centres of the brain, potentially creating a craving that the subject perceives as internally generated. They wake up wanting a specific soda, believing it is their own idea, not realising it was a planted suggestion. This is a violation of cognitive liberty at the very least.

Then there is the issue of data privacy. The devices that enable these interventions are sophisticated surveillance tools. To time the sound cues correctly, they must monitor brainwaves, heart rate, movement, and potentially even verbal mutterings (somniloquy). This creates a biometric blueprint of the sleeper's most vulnerable moments. Who owns this data? If you use a free app to incubate creativity, does the developer own the resulting dream patterns? Can they sell your sleep architecture to an insurance company, who might deny you coverage because your lack of deep sleep suggests a risk of Alzheimer's? Can they sell your emotional reactivity data to a political campaign? The bedroom is the place where we are most naked, physically and neurologically. If the Terms of Service of our sleep devices allow for data harvesting, we are effectively installing a spy in our own heads.

Beyond manipulation and surveillance, there is the risk of addiction. This is the Holodeck problem; as lucid dreaming technology becomes more effective and immersive, the contrast between the waking world and the dream world will sharpen. Real life is hard. It is full of grief, boredom, physical limitations, and consequences. The engineered dream world is a place of god-like power, infinite pleasure, and zero consequence. If you can fly through the cosmos, reunite with lost loved ones, and satisfy every desire in a lucid dream, why would you want to wake up?

We might see the emergence of somniphilia or reality rejection, where individuals choose to spend as much time as possible in chemically or technologically assisted sleep. The programmable sanctuary could become a programmable coffin (and we have seen this in movies and TV shows), a place where we retreat from the difficulties of human existence into a perfect, solipsistic loop. This attrition of engagement with the real world is a profound existential risk. A society of lucid dreamers might be a society that stops trying to fix reality because they have a better alternative asleep.

Furthermore, there is the philosophical question of the value of the unknown. Dream engineering assumes that we know what our dreams should be. We assume that a good dream is a happy one, or a productive one, or a lucid one. We try to sanitise the night, removing the nightmares and the anxiety. But evolutionary biologists argue that the bad dreams serve a purpose. The chaos, the fear, and the randomness of un-engineered sleep are likely essential for emotional regulation. They are the brain's way of running threat simulations and processing negative emotions. By continually intervening to make our sleep productive or pleasant, we might be stunting our own emotional growth. We might be creating a generation of people who are fragile because they have never faced their demons in the safety of the dark.

Finally, we must consider the issue of consent and power dynamics. Who controls the device? In a domestic abuse scenario, a partner could theoretically misuse sleep-learning technology to reinforce dependency or fear while the victim sleeps. In a military context, soldiers could be programmed for aggression or desensitised to trauma during their rest cycles. The technology is neutral, but its application is bound only by the ethics of the user.

As we stand on the precipice of this new era, we need something akin to a Bill of Rights for the sleeping mind. We need legislation that defines the neuro-privacy of the citizen. This might include the Right to Non-Interference, which is the legal guarantee that no third party can introduce stimuli into a person's sleep without their explicit, informed, and revocable consent. It might include a ban on commercial advertising in dream incubation technologies or hardware we have in the bedroom.

The programmable sanctuary we have built throughout this book is a tool for health and recovery. It is designed to support the sleeper, not to exploit them. But as with all powerful tools, the difference between medicine and poison is in the dosage and the intent.

We have spent centuries fighting for freedom of speech and freedom of thought. In the coming decades, the battlefront will shift inward. We will have to fight for freedom of sleep. We must ensure that the dream remains a wild, protected space, a national park of the subconscious, rather than a billboard or a factory floor. The ultimate goal of engineering dreams should be to give us the strength to face our waking lives, not to replace them. The night belongs to the dreamer, and it must stay that way.

8

Executive Function

ARIANNA HUFFINGTON

Sleep as Logistics

For generations, the corporate and political elite have worn sleep deprivation as a badge of honour. The archetype of the titan of industry or Prime Minister of note was someone who slept four hours a night, answered emails at 3am, and treated rest as a regrettable biological weakness. The implicit message was clear: sleep is for the weak. If you are sleeping, you are losing. Time spent unconscious is time not spent trading, negotiating, or leading (or being seen to be leading).

This narrative is not only scientifically illiterate; it is professionally dangerous. In high-stakes environments, whether that is a boardroom during a merger, a hospital operating theatre, or a military command post, the primary asset being leveraged is the decision-making capability of the leader. When an executive sleeps for four hours, their cognitive supply chain breaks down. We know from decades of research that sleep deprivation specifically targets the prefrontal cortex; the CEO of the brain. This is the area responsible for executive function, impulse control, complex analysis, and emotional regulation. When a leader is under-slept, they do not lose their ability to speak or perform basic tasks. They lose their ability to handle nuance. They become more reactive, more prone to bias, less empathetic, and more likely to make high-risk decisions for short-term gain.

Therefore, we need to completely reframe how we view rest. We must stop viewing sleep as a lifestyle luxury, something you do if you have time after the work is done. We must start viewing sleep as an operational requirement, as critical as the fuel in a jet or the charge in a server battery. In a logistics framework, sleep is an inventory management problem. You start the day with a certain amount of cognitive capital. Every decision you make, every email you filter, every emotion you regulate depletes that capital. Sleep is the only biological process that restocks the warehouse. If you consistently ship more product (decisions) than you restock (sleep), you enter a state of deficit. In finance, this leads to bankruptcy and in corporate leadership, it leads to burnout and catastrophic error.

The most effective leaders of the modern era are shifting to this athlete mindset. A Formula One team does not let their driver party all night before a race. They manage the driver's recovery with the same precision they manage the car's telemetry. They know that a 1 per cent drop in reaction time is the difference between winning and crashing. Corporate athletes are beginning to apply the same rigour. This operational approach changes the scheduling dynamic. In the old model, sleep got whatever time was left over. In the logistics model, sleep is priority number 1.

This means protecting the sleep window with the same ferocity used to protect a meeting with a key investor. If a flight lands at 11pm and there is a meeting at 7am, the logistics-minded leader recognises this as a risk factor. They might push the meeting back, not because they are tired, but because they know their cognitive inventory will be too low to deliver value. They are protecting the asset. This framework also de-personalises the issue. When a team member says, 'I need to rest', it shouldn't be heard as a complaint. It should be heard as a status report: 'My battery is at 5 per cent; I need to recharge to function'. This removes the stigma and moves the conversation from toughness to readiness.

In the military, this is already doctrine. Fatigue Management is a core component of mission planning. Commanders are taught that a tired soldier is a liability. They implement sleep banking strategies before operations and enforced rest cycles during them. They understand that courage cannot compensate for a brain that has stopped processing visual data correctly.

For the corporate executive, 'Sleep as Logistics' involves three key shifts:

1. **Quantification:** You cannot manage what you do not measure. Just as you track revenue and burn rate, you must track recovery. This is where the wearable tech discussed in Chapter 2 becomes a professional tool. A leader should know their average sleep score. If they are trending down, it is a signal to de-load the schedule, just as a drop in sales is a signal to adjust strategy.

2. **Defensive Scheduling:** This means building buffers around the sleep window. It involves setting a hard digital sunset for the team, establishing that emails sent after a certain hour will not be answered until morning. This protects the leader's own winding-down process and prevents the always-on anxiety that destroys sleep quality.

3. **The Nap as a Tactical Weapon:** In the logistics model, a twenty-minute nap is not laziness; it is a system reboot. It is a strategic intervention to clear adenosine (sleep pressure) and restore vigilance. A leader closing their door for twenty minutes at 2pm is not checking out; they are ensuring they are sharp for the 4pm negotiation.

The stakes are too high for the sleepless hero myth man to survive. The problems leaders face today are not algorithmic;

they cannot be solved by brute force and long hours. They are heuristic; they require insight, creativity, and emotional intelligence. These are the very faculties that sleep deprivation destroys first. To treat sleep as logistics is to acknowledge reality. The biology of the human being has not changed in fifty thousand years. The leader who respects their sleep is not doing so to be comfortable; they are doing so to be dangerous. They are ensuring that when the crisis comes, when the market crashes, or when the competitor attacks, they are the most awake person in the room. And in a world of exhausted zombies, the awake person is king.

Travel Protocols

For the modern executive, travel is often glamourised as a perk of the job. But biologically, crossing time zones is an act of violence against the circadian system. Jet lag is not merely being tired. It is a fundamental physiological desynchrony. Your liver, your heart, your brain, and your gut are all running on different clocks. The master clock in the brain (the Suprachiasmatic Nucleus) knows it is daylight, but the liver thinks it is 3am and is unprepared to process food. The result is circadian misalignment, a state characterised by cognitive fog, digestive distress, immune suppression, and profound mood instability. I have experienced this more than I care to remember; and it is a standard cost of living in Australia and travelling globally to where the projects and clients are.

When the stakes are high (when you are landing in London to close a deal or arriving in Tokyo to manage a crisis) you cannot afford this biological lag. You need a protocol. You need to treat the flight not as a passive waiting period, but as an active phase of circadian engineering. People would pay good money if someone just solved jet lag with a medication (me included)!

The first rule of the travel protocol is to understand the two most powerful Zeitgebers (time-givers) that reset the human clock: Light and Food. Most travellers manage these incorrectly. They eat when the plane gives them food and sleep when the movie ends. This is a recipe for disaster. To beat jet lag, you must decouple your behaviour from the airline's schedule and align it with the destination.

The most underutilised lever for overcoming jet lag is the stomach. Research suggests that while light resets the master clock in the brain, food resets the peripheral clocks in the organs. If you eat a heavy meal at what your body thinks is 2am, you are confirming to your liver that it is still the middle of the night (or rather, a strange time to be eating), anchoring your metabolic clock to your home time zone.

The *Argonaut* protocol, derived from military and CIA studies, suggests a strategic fast. The goal is to suspend the metabolic clock during transit.

- **The Tactic:** Stop eating as soon as you get to the airport. Drink only water and electrolytes during the flight. This signals a scarcity state to the body, which makes the circadian system more fluid and adaptable.

- **The Restart:** Break the fast with a high-protein breakfast at the *correct breakfast time* of your destination. This massive caloric signal acts as a starting gun. It tells every cell in your body: 'The day has begun. This is morning'.

Light is the primary drug. It suppresses melatonin and drives wakefulness. But its effect depends entirely on when you see it. This is known as the Phase Response Curve.

- **Eastward Travel (The Hard Shift):** Flying New York to London (advancing the clock). You are trying to make your body wake up earlier. You need to seek light in the early morning of the destination and strictly avoid light in the late evening.
  - *The Mistake:* Landing in London at 10am and wearing sunglasses. No. You need those photons to hit your retina to push your clock forward.
  - *The Mistake:* Using a laptop at 10pm London time. This light tells your brain it is still afternoon in New York, pushing your clock the wrong way (delaying it).
- **Westward Travel (The Easy Shift):** Flying London to New York (delaying the clock). You are trying to stay awake later. You need to seek light in the late afternoon/ evening.
  - *The Tactic:* Go for a walk in the sunlight upon arrival. Keep the hotel lights bright until 10pm local time. This pushes the sleep gate later.

Melatonin is widely misunderstood, and most people take huge doses (5mg or 10mg) right before bed as a sedative (yes, I am guilty of doing this on long haul flights). This often leads to grogginess and vivid dreams. For travel, melatonin should be used as a 'chronobiotic' a time-shifting drug.

- **Dose:** Low. 0.5mg to 3mg is sufficient.
- **Timing:** For Eastward travel, take it in the late afternoon or early evening of the destination time, assuming you can sleep. This signals the brain that darkness is coming earlier than expected, pulling the sleep window forward.

The airplane cabin is an engine of dehydration and fatigue. Generally the air pressure is equivalent to standing on top of an 8,000-foot mountain, and the humidity is lower than the Sahara Desert.

- **Hydration:** The rule is 250ml of water for every hour of flying. No alcohol. Alcohol is a sedative, not a sleep aid. It destroys REM sleep and dehydrates the brain, compounding the jet lag.
- **The Micro-Climate:** Create a portable sanctuary. Noise-cancelling headphones are mandatory to lower the sonic load on the brain. A contoured sleep mask (that allows eye movement) ensures total darkness even if the person next to you opens their shade.

There is one scenario where you ignore all of the above: the trip that lasts less than 48 hours. If you are flying from Los

Angeles to New York for a single meeting and returning the next day, do not adapt.

- **The Tactic:** Keep your watch on Los Angeles time. If the meeting is at 9am NY time, that is 6am LA time which is painful but manageable. When the meeting ends at 5pm NY time (2pm LA time), do not go out for dinner. Go to the hotel, close the blackout curtains, and sleep on your home schedule.
- **The Logic:** It takes about one day to adjust one hour of time difference. It is physiologically impossible to adapt to a three-hour shift in 24 hours. Trying to adapt will only leave you in circadian limbo. It is better to be a fully functioning Californian in New York than a broken biological hybrid.

The moment you enter the hotel room, the mission changes. You must sanitise the environment (discussed in the next section), but you must also signal safety to the body.

- **Thermoregulation:** A hot shower or bath upon arrival is not just for hygiene. It dilates the blood vessels. When you step out into the cooler air, your core body temperature drops rapidly. This drop mimics the natural temperature dip that occurs at sleep onset, tricking the body into feeling tired.
- **Grounding:** High-stakes travel is stressful and cortisol is high. If possible, do 20 minutes of moderate exercise; e.g. a light jog or yoga. This burns off the accumulated

adrenaline of the travel day and increases adenosine pressure for the coming night.

Ultimately, managing travel is about discipline. It requires saying no to the free Champagne and cocktails and chef made dinners in business class. It requires forcing yourself to walk outside in the sunlight when your body is screaming for a nap. But the payoff is performance. The executive who lands with a synchronised clock is the executive who notices the nuance in the contract that the exhausted counterparty misses. I also swear by compression socks.

The Hotel Environment

The modern hotel room is a paradox. It is marketed as a sanctuary of luxury and rest, sold on the thread count of the sheets and the thickness of the mattress. Yet, for the average human being, it is often a hostile environment as it is an unfamiliar cave. I never sleep well on the first night in a hotel room when I am travelling alone and my troubles can be explained by evolutionary biology; it is a phenomenon known as the 'First Night Effect'. When humans sleep in a new environment, one hemisphere of the brain stays in a state of higher vigilance (essentially half-awake) to scan for predators. This is not anxiety; it is a hard-coded survival mechanism. You are vulnerable, and your brain refuses to fully off-line until it is sure the cave is safe.

To rest effectively when the stakes are high, you cannot simply hope the hotel is good. You must actively engineer the space.

You must hack the room to neutralise the threats and signal safety to the amygdala. This requires a 'Hotel Audit' protocol, executed the moment you drop your bags.

Hotel designers are obsessed with ambient lighting, which is disastrous for sleep. The room is often filled with vampire light from the standby LED on the television, the glowing green display of the smoke detector, the blue light of the digital clock, and the light leaking from the hallway under the door.

- **The Kit:** The seasoned traveller never travels without a roll of black electrical tape or a pack of blocking stickers.
- **The Protocol:** Spend two minutes taping over every LED in the room. Unplug the digital clock or face it to the wall.
- **The Curtain Gap:** Most hotel curtains do not close flush. They leave a 'light dagger' a vertical strip of street-lamp glare that cuts across the room.
  - *The Hack:* Use the clips on the trousers hangers found in the closet to clamp the curtains shut. In a pinch, a safety pin or even a hair clip works.
- **The Door:** The hallway is always bright. Roll up a bath towel and jam it against the base of the door. This blocks the light leak and also dampens the sound of footsteps.

Hotels are acoustically porous. You are at the mercy of the elevator ding, the ice machine, the plumbing of the room above, and the late-night habits of the guest next door. The silence of a hotel room is rarely true silence; it is a waiting game for the next noise.

- **The Defence:** Do not rely on earplugs alone, as they can amplify internal body sounds (heartbeat) and cause anxiety. Instead, build a sonic wall.
- **The Tool:** Use a portable white noise machine or a dedicated app on your phone connected to a Bluetooth speaker.
- **The Setting:** You want Brown Noise (lower frequency, rumble) rather than White Noise (high frequency, hiss). Brown noise masks low-frequency thuds (doors slamming) more effectively. Place the speaker near the source of the noise (usually the door or the window) to scramble the incoming sound waves before they reach the bed.

To defeat the First Night Effect, you need to trick the brain into thinking it is at home. This is where olfactory (smell) and tactile cues become critical.

- **Scent:** The olfactory bulb has a direct hotline to the limbic system (emotion and memory). If you use a specific pillow spray (like lavender or cedarwood) at home, bring a travel-sized bottle. Spraying the hotel pillow with a home scent sends a powerful chemical signal of safety to the brain, overriding the new cave alarm.
- **Touch:** Hotel pillows are a gamble as they are often too high (neck strain) or too soft (suffocation). If space per-

mits, pack your own pillowcase (I always travel with my own pillow for long haul flight and hotel sleep optimisation). The texture and smell of your own fabric against your face is a potent subconscious reassurance.

Finally, you cannot sleep deep if you do not feel safe. The subconscious mind is tracking the door.

- **The Lock:** Always engage the deadbolt and the swinging security latch.
- **The Wedge:** For high-stakes or high-risk travel, a simple rubber door wedge adds a mechanical layer of security that allows the brain to stand down. Knowing that the door physically cannot open from the outside removes a layer of vigilance.

The goal of the hotel hack is to standardise the variable. You cannot control the city, the time zone, or the quality of the mattress. But by controlling the light, the sound, the temperature, and the security, you create a micro-environment that is consistent, predictable, and conducive to recovery.

Crisis Management

There are moments in professional life when the standard rules of sleep hygiene do not apply. A server farm crashes at 2am, a major cyber incident occurs, or a merger deal enters the final, bruising week of due diligence. In these scenarios, the goal is no longer optimal health or perfect sleep. The goal is simply to maintain cognitive function above the threshold of catastrophic error. This is survival mode. Most people handle a crisis by attempting to power through. They drink excessive amounts of coffee, eat sugar, and try to stay awake until the job is done. This is a tactical mistake. The brain is not a machine that can run indefinitely on adrenaline; it is a biological organ that accumulates toxic waste products (adenosine) the longer it is awake. After roughly seventeen hours of wakefulness, your cognitive performance is equivalent to having a blood alcohol concentration of 0.05 per cent. After twenty-four hours, it is 0.10 per cent aka legally drunk. In a crisis, you are essentially making critical decisions while intoxicated.

To survive a crisis without crashing, you need a protocol for 'Operational Rest'. This is a militarised approach to sleep, treating it as a resource to be snatched in calculated bursts. If continuous operations are required over several days, you must protect a core anchor of sleep. The absolute biological floor for maintaining executive function is roughly four hours (two full ninety-minute sleep cycles plus transition time). This anchor sleep should ideally happen at the same time every twenty-four-hour period, preferably during the circadian trough between 2am and 6am, when the body's drive for sleep is highest and the urge to be awake is lowest. Sleeping four hours is not sustainable long-term, but for a three-to-five-day crisis window, it acts as a firewall against psychosis and total collapse. It allows the brain to complete the essential wash cycle of the glymphatic system, clearing enough toxins to allow for function the next day.

When you cannot get four hours, you must nap. But you must nap with mathematical precision. There are only two safe durations for a crisis nap: twenty minutes or ninety minutes.

- **The Power Nap (20 Minutes):** This is a Stage 2 nap. It provides a burst of alertness and clears the immediate pressure of adenosine without letting the brain sink into deep, slow-wave sleep. You wake up sharp.
- **The Cycle Nap (90 Minutes):** This allows for a full sleep cycle, including REM. It aids emotional regulation and creative problem-solving.
- **The Danger Zone (30 to 60 Minutes):** You must avoid waking up in this window at all costs. If you sleep for forty-five minutes, you will likely wake up from deep sleep. You will suffer from sleep inertia, you know what that feels like, it's that heavy, groggy, disoriented feeling where your limbs feel like lead and your brain feels like it is underwater. In a crisis, sleep inertia is dangerous. It can take thirty minutes to shake off, rendering you useless when you are needed most. If you only have forty-five minutes, do not sleep. Meditate or rest your eyes, but do not cross the threshold.

Caffeine is often misused in a crisis as a replacement for sleep. It should be used as a force multiplier for sleep. The most effective protocol is the 'Nappuccino'.

1. Drink a cup of black coffee quickly (cool it down with an ice cube).

2. Immediately lie down and close your eyes for a twenty-minute nap.
3. The caffeine takes about twenty minutes to cross the blood-brain barrier and hit the adenosine receptors.
4. You wake up at the exact moment the caffeine kicks in, having also cleared some adenosine through sleep. You get a double-spike of alertness without the grogginess.

The best way to handle a crisis is to prepare for it before it starts. If you know a high-intensity period is coming such as the end of the quarter, a planned surgery, a military operation etc., you should engage in 'prophylactic napping'. Studies have shown that subjects who extended their sleep to nine or ten hours a night for a week before a period of sleep deprivation performed significantly better than those who entered the crisis with a normal sleep debt. You can literally 'bank' rest. It acts as a cognitive buffer. If you anticipate a sleepless week, spend the weekend prior sleeping as much as possible.

In a 24-hour operation, light is your primary control switch. If you are working through the night, you must saturate your environment with bright, blue-enriched light. This suppresses melatonin and tricks the clock. However, when it is time for your anchor sleep or your ninety-minute nap, you must achieve total blackout darkness. Wear a mask. The contrast is key. The brain needs a binary signal: It is FULL DAY (work) or It is FULL NIGHT (rest). Twilight is the enemy of alertness.

When the crisis breaks, do not attempt to pay back the sleep debt in one massive twenty-hour coma. This will cause *social jet lag* and throw your clock off for the coming week. Instead, go to bed early (say, 9pm) for the next three nights and allow yourself to wake up naturally. Do not set an alarm if possible. Focus on sleep efficiency; dark, cool, and quiet. Your deep sleep percentage will naturally rebound (a phenomenon called REM rebound) as the brain aggressively prioritises the stages it missed.

In crisis management, perfection is not the goal; the goal is to avoid the lethal combination of fatigue and hubris. By adhering to the protocols of anchor sleep, precise napping, and tactical caffeine, you accept your biological limitations while maximising your remaining capacity. You survive the storm not by ignoring the need for rest, but by engineering it.

Organisational Culture

We have spent much of this book discussing the hardware and software of sleep i.e. sensors, mattresses, lighting, and biological protocols. But the single biggest disruptor of sleep in the modern world is not blue light or caffeine: It is culture. It is the unwritten, invisible contract that suggests presence equals productivity and that rest is a form of disengagement.

In many high-performance organisations and toxic work places, there is a pervasive cult of the sleepless. It is signalled in subtle ways: the email sent at 11pm that gets a 'thumbs up' from the boss; the boasting about pulling an all-nighter to finish a deck; the side-eye given to the employee who leaves at 5pm. These signals create a psychological environment where sleep is viewed as a career liability.

The result is a workforce that is perpetually tired but wired. They are physically present but cognitively degraded. They are suffering from *presenteeism*; sitting in the chair, moving the mouse, but lacking the executive function to do deep, creative work. For the organisation, this is a silent haemorrhage of value. It leads to higher error rates, lower emotional intelligence, higher turnover, and a stagnation of innovation.

To fix this, we cannot just tell employees to sleep more. We have to engineer the culture to make rest possible. We must therefore move from a culture of always being switched on to a culture of oscillating engagement; high intensity followed by high recovery. The tip of the spear in this cultural shift is the *Right to Disconnect*. Originally a legislative concept emerging in Europe and now spreading globally, it protects the employee from being penalised for refusing to answer work communications outside of working hours. However, for a company, simply following the law is not enough. The policy must be woven into the cultural fabric of the team. It requires a hard reset on the expected response time. In a hyper-connected world, we have defaulted to an expectation of immediacy. If I Slack or text message you, I expect an answer now. If I email you, I expect a reply within the hour.

This constant scanning for notifications prevents the brain from entering the default mode network; the state of rest and wandering that is essential for recovery. It keeps the cortisol drip turned on 24/7. A sleep-smart organisation implements batch processing protocols. They establish that email is an asynchronous medium. Unless a message is marked URGENT (a tag that should be used sparingly and with good grace), the expectation is that it will be answered within 24 hours, not 24 minutes. This gives employees the psychological permission to close their laptops and, crucially, to turn off their phones in the evening without the fear of missing a crisis.

Culture is not what you write in the handbook; it is what the leadership does (do as I do, not as I say). If a CEO stands on stage and talks about mental health, but then sends non-urgent emails to their team at 2am, the culture is 2am. The team looks at the timestamp, not the handbook. They interpret the late email as a signal: This is how you succeed here.

To change this, leaders must practise loud leaving and scheduled sending.

- **Scheduled Sending:** If an executive is working late (perhaps because that suits their personal chronotype), they should use the schedule send feature to ensure the email arrives in the employee's inbox at 8:30am the next morning, not at midnight. This protects the employee's evening while allowing the leader to work when they want.
- **Loud Leaving:** Leaders should visibly disconnect. They should say, I am logging off now to rest, and then actually stay offline. They need to role-model the

boundary. When the team sees that the boss prioritises recovery, the stigma of rest dissolves.

In safety-critical industries like aviation, mining, and trucking, fatigue is not treated as a morale issue; it is treated as a hazard, just like a toxic chemical or a slippery floor. These industries use Fatigue Risk Management Systems (FRMS) within Health and Safety (HSE) frameworks to quantify and mitigate the risk.

White-collar organisations are beginning to adopt this mindset. They are acknowledging that a fatigued trader, surgeon, or coder is a safety risk to the business. They are implementing fatigue audits of their workflows. For example, does the team in London have to wake up at 4am for a weekly call with the team in Sydney? Or can the meeting time rotate so the pain is shared? Is the deal team being forced to work three weekends in a row? If so, the FRMS flags this as a red zone risk and mandates a compulsory recovery day. This moves the conversation from Are you tough enough? to Are you safe enough?

We are seeing a physical manifestation of this culture shift in the return of the rest pod. For years, nap pods in tech offices were dismissed as gimmicks or performative perks. But as the science of the power nap becomes undeniable, companies are reinstalling them as essential infrastructure. However, the pod is useless without the cultural permission to use it. If an employee fears they will be judged for sleeping at 2pm, the pod will stay empty. The culture must reframe the nap. It is not sleeping on the job; it is system maintenance. Some companies are even rebranding them as recharge stations or focus rooms to bypass the lazy stigma. The message is: go in there for twenty minutes so you can come out and crush the afternoon.

Finally, organisations are beginning to respect the biological diversity of their workforce. As we discussed in earlier chapters, larks (morning types) and owls (evening types) have different peak performance windows. A rigid 9-to-5 structure forces the owl to wake up during their biological night and forces the lark to keep working when their brain has shut down. A chronotype-aware culture allows for flex-scheduling. It lets the larks start at 7am and leave at 3pm. It lets the owls start at 11am and work until 7pm. By aligning the work schedule with the biological clock, the organisation gets more productivity per hour, and the employee gets better sleep. What a culture shift this would be!

The argument for this cultural revolution is ultimately economic. The cost of burnout is astronomical across western corporate productivity. It is measured in sick days, in health insurance claims, workplace accidents, in then in recruitment fees to replace staff who quit, and in the phantom cost of poor decision-making. Some clients ask for employee turnover rates as an indicator of risk, so this is something every leader should be considering. A company that respects sleep is a company that is playing the long game. They are building a sustainable human capital strategy. They understand that you cannot burn the candle at both ends forever. By implementing the right to disconnect, modelling healthy boundaries, and treating fatigue as a manageable risk, they create a culture where high performance is sustainable.

In this environment, the employee who says, I'm going home to sleep, is not checking out. They are preparing to win. They are protecting the asset. And the organisation that supports them is the one that will survive the marathon of the modern economy.

9

The Sleep Data Ecosystem

> Surveillance capitalism claims human experience as free raw material for translation into behavioural data.
>
> SHOSHANA ZUBOFF

The Data Ecosystem

Every morning, millions of people perform a new secular ritual. Before they kiss their partner, brush their teeth, or even fully open their eyes, they reach for their phone. They open an app, wait for a spinning wheel to complete its rotation, and then stare at a number. A Sleep Score. A Readiness Index. A Body Battery percentage.

For the user, this interaction is the end of the story. The device on their wrist or finger has spoken, delivering a verdict on their night. But from a technological perspective, that number is not the end; it is merely the surface of a vast, invisible ocean. The journey that your biological data takes; from the pulse in your wrist to the server farm in a distant arctic desert, is a complex odyssey through the Data Ecosystem. Understanding this map is the first step in understanding who truly owns the night (and your peace of mind).

The journey begins at the edge of the network: your body. Whether it is an Apple Watch, an Oura Ring, a Whoop strap, or a Withings mattress mat, the device is technically known as a peripheral. Contrary to popular belief, these devices are rarely sending raw data in real-time. The bandwidth required to transmit millisecond-by-millisecond data packets would drain the tiny battery in minutes. Instead, the device acts as a data compression engine. It processes the data locally, like an edge computing system. Its internal processor analyses the raw noise of your movement and blood flow, strips away the static, and calculates summary metrics: heart rate, variability, temperature deviation. It stores these summaries in its flash memory, waiting for the digital handshake connection.

The moment you open the app on your phone, a connection is forged. This is done via Bluetooth Low Energy (BLE), a protocol designed to sip power while moving small packets of data. This is also a critical vulnerability point for cyber risk. Whilst modern encryption standards are robust, the handshake moment; when the device pairs with the phone, can theoretically be sniffed by malicious actors in close proximity. However, don't worry; in the domestic ecosystem, the real transfer is mundane: the device dumps its memory buffer into the smartphone.

Once the data hits your phone, it enters the most critical phase of its existence: aggregation. In the early days of wearables, data lived in silos. Your Fitbit data lived in the Fitbit app; your meditation data lived in Headspace. They never spoke to each other. Today, the landscape is dominated by two Leviathans: Apple Health (HealthKit) and Google Health Connect. These are not apps; they are infrastructure. They act as the central switchboard for the human body's data downloads. When you set up your sleep tracker, you almost certainly clicked 'Allow' on a permission screen asking to 'Write Data to Health'. This grants your tracker permission to deposit its findings into the central encrypted vault of the operating system.

This hub model is powerful as it allows for inter-app triangulation. A nutrition app can read your sleep data from the hub to recommend a breakfast. A fitness app can read your recovery score to suggest a workout. The phone becomes a digital medical record, updated every second. Apple, in particular, emphasises that this data is encrypted on-device and, if you use iCloud, encrypted in transit and at rest, meaning even

Apple technically cannot read it (NB: if your Advanced Data Protection setting is enabled).

However, the data does not just stay on your phone. Simultaneously, the companion app (the Oura app, the Fitbit app) is sending a copy of that data out to the wider internet. It travels via Wi-Fi or cellular networks to the Cloud. The Cloud is a euphemism for a physical computer owned by someone else. Usually, it is a server rack sitting in a data centre in Virginia or Ireland, rented from Amazon Web Services (AWS), Microsoft Azure, or Google Cloud Platform.

This is where the proprietary magic happens. The raw metrics are run through the company's black box algorithms. This is where your Sleep Score is actually calculated. The company compares your data against their massive historical dataset (the population norm) to give you context.

This step is the divergence point for ownership. Once your data is on their server, it is subject to their Terms of Service. In most cases, you own the data, but you grant them a 'perpetual, worldwide, royalty-free licence' to use it for service improvement and research. This legal loophole effectively makes them the co-owners of your biology.

The ecosystem expands further through Application Programming Interfaces (APIs), this is the web of connections that allows third-party services to plug into your data stream. Consider a corporate wellness program. Your employer offers you a discount on health insurance if you walk 10,000 steps and sleep 7 hours. To get the discount, you link your tracker to the insurance company's app and you do this via an API. You are creating a permanent pipe from the proprietary cloud to the insurance company's cloud.

Or consider coaching services these AI apps that ingest your sleep data to give you advice. They pull data from the API, process it on *their* servers (often using OpenAI or other LLMs), and send the advice back.

Beneath this visible flow of useful data lies the shadow ecosystem. This involves data brokers. While reputable hardware companies (like Apple or Oura) generally do not sell identifiable user data to brokers, the free apps in the ecosystem often do. That free snore recorder app or that smart alarm app? Its business model is likely not the app; it is you. It collects behavioural data, e.g. what time you go to bed, what time you wake up, your location history, and sells anonymised bundles to data aggregators. These aggregators build profiles of consumers.

They know that *User XYZ123* sleeps poorly on Sundays (anxiety), wakes up at 5am (high achiever or shift worker), and lives in a high-income postal/zip code. This profile is then sold to advertisers. Suddenly, you start seeing ads for sedatives or luxury mattresses. You are not just a user; you are a 'sleep phenotype' being auctioned off to the highest bidder.

The final element of the ecosystem is time. How long does the data live? In the old analog world, medical records were paper in a filing cabinet that could burn or be shredded. In the digital ecosystem, data has potentially infinite persistence.

Your sleep data from five years ago still exists on a server somewhere. It is a permanent biological record of your past self. This longevity is a double-edged sword. It is incredible for tracking long-term health trends. But it is also a liability. If you run for political office in ten years, could a leak of your sleep data reveal a period of erratic behaviour or insomnia that suggests instability? If you apply for life insurance, could your decade of 'low deep sleep' be used to predict Alzheimer's risk and deny you a policy?

The ecosystem is efficient, interconnected, and miraculous; it allows for the quantified self to exist. But it is also leaky, vast, and fundamentally outside the user's physical control. We feed the machine our most intimate moments; our dreams, our tossing and turning, our heartbeats in the dark, and in return, it gives us a graph. The question to ask is: is that a fair trade? And as the ecosystem grows, how do we ensure that we remain the owners of the map, rather than just the terrain being mapped?

Privacy and Surveillance

In the 20th century, the ultimate invasion of privacy was the wiretap. It was the fear that someone, somewhere, was listening to your conversations. In the 21st century, the wiretap has been replaced by the biosensor, and the conversation being listened to is the silent dialogue between your nervous system and your heart.

We have built a 'Glass Bedroom' from a data perspective. By inviting connected sensors into our sleep, we have turned the most private act of human existence into a broadcast. While we focus on the benefits such as the optimised recovery and the early warning systems for illness, we rarely stop to consider who is tuning into the signal. The reality is that sleep data is a new form of currency, and there is a thriving, largely unregulated market that trades in the futures of your fatigue.

The first line of defence offered by tech companies is anonymisation. They claim that while they collect your data, they strip away your name, email, and social security number before sharing it with researchers or partners. They sell trends, not people.

This is a comforting but could be fiction; in the world of big data, true anonymity is mathematically impossible. Researchers have repeatedly demonstrated a phenomenon known as the Mosaic Effect. By combining a sanitised dataset (like sleep patterns) with an external dataset (like public geolocation logs or social media timestamps), it is easier than might make you comfortable to re-identify individuals.

Your sleep pattern is as unique as a fingerprint. If a data broker has a dataset showing a user who wakes up at 5:30am in a specific suburb, goes for a run (GPS data), and then drives to a specific office building, they don't need a name tag. They know who you are. The data collected by a free sleep tracking app (which creates a revenue stream by selling these de-identified bundles to aggregators) can be reverse-engineered to build a granular dossier of your life. They know when you are sleeping, when you are intimate, and when you are awake and vulnerable to a late-night impulse purchase.

The surveillance of sleep is moving aggressively into the workplace. For decades, employers monitored productivity via inputs: time cards, keystrokes, and badge swipes. Now, they are monitoring capacity. This often arrives in the guise of benevolence: the corporate wellness program, or a company hands out free Fitbits or Oura rings to its staff. They launch a challenge: 'Sleep for seven hours a night and earn points towards lower health insurance premiums!' It sounds like a win-win. The employee gets a toy and a discount; the employer gets a healthier, more productive workforce.

But this transaction breaks the biological firewall between the professional and the personal. When you sync your tracker with your employer's wellness platform, you are potentially giving them visibility into your off-hours behaviour. Consider the promotion scenario from hell. Two candidates are up for a high-stress executive role. Both are qualified, but the wellness dashboard shows that Candidate A averages eight hours of stable, deep sleep, while Candidate B averages five hours of fragmented, chaotic sleep. Does the company subconsciously (or explicitly) view Candidate B as a burnout risk? Is Candidate B passed over not because of their performance, but because of their physiology?

This creates a new form of discrimination: Bio-profiling. We have laws preventing discrimination based on gender, race, and disability. We do not yet have laws preventing discrimination based on sleep architecture. In a hyper-competitive economy, your sleep score could become a metric on your annual performance review. The boss isn't just watching you work; they are watching you rest to ensure you are working on your recharging efficiency.

The deepest risk, however, is not what the data shows, but what it implies. This is the power of inference. Machine learning algorithms are pattern recognition engines. They can spot correlations that are invisible to human doctors. Sleep data is incredibly leak-prone regarding health status. Changes in sleep architecture often precede the diagnosis of major diseases by years.

- **Mental Health:** A sudden shift in REM latency (how quickly you enter dreams) is a strong predictor of onsite depression.
- **Neurology:** People with 'REM Sleep Behaviour Disorder' (acting out dreams) have a extremely high probability of developing Parkinson's disease or Lewy Body Dementia within a decade.
- **Pregnancy:** Shifts in resting heart rate and body temperature during the night can detect pregnancy as early as five days after conception; often before the woman herself knows.

This leads to the Target story being repeated: Years ago, the retailer Target infamously predicted a teenager was pregnant based on her shopping habits and sent coupons for baby clothes to her house, alerting her father (whose loyalty card it was). Today, that prediction can be made based on sleep data. If a third-party app (say, a period tracker or a sleep recorder) detects these patterns, who do they tell? Do they sell that 'high probability pregnancy' tag to advertisers selling baby formula? Do they sell the 'early onset depression' tag to pharmaceutical companies advertising antidepressants?

Even more terrifying is the insurance angle. Life insurance and health insurance rely on risk assessment. Currently, they use blunt indicator tools: age, BMI, smoker status. Imagine if they had access to the 'inference layer'. A life insurer could buy a dataset, run an algorithm, and identify that *User XYZ123* has a sleep signature consistent with early Alzheimer's. They could then raise that user's premiums or deny coverage entirely, long before a doctor has written a formal diagnosis. The user is penalised for a disease they don't even know they might have yet.

Finally, we must consider the military and security implications. In 2018, the fitness tracking app Strava released a 'global heatmap' showing where its users were running. Internet sleuths immediately noticed bright lines of activity in the middle of deserts in Syria and Afghanistan. Soldiers wearing Fitbits had unwittingly mapped out the perimeters of secret US military bases. Sleep data poses a similar risk. A sudden disruption in the sleep patterns of key government officials, diplomats, or CEOs could signal a crisis before it becomes public news. If the CEO of a major public company suddenly stops sleeping, or their heart rate variability crashes, it is a signal of extreme stress. To a hedge fund trader, that data is insider information. It suggests a pending scandal, a failed merger, or a bad earnings report.

If hackers were to breach the servers of a major sleep tracking company, they wouldn't just get email addresses. They would get the biological fingerprint of the elite. They would know exactly when the President is in deep sleep and unable to respond to a phone call. They would know which general is exhausted and prone to error. Biology as a vector for national security; who would have thought it?

The ultimate consequence of this surveillance is psychological. When we know we are being watched, we change our behaviours accordingly (or at least we try). We perform like trained seals. If we know our insurance depends on our sleep score, we lie in bed anxious about the score, which destroys the sleep. If we know our boss is checking our perceived readiness, we might strap the watch to the dog to fake a good night's rest. It reminds me of an episode of Dr Who when all the humans had to walk around with smiles on their faces pretending to be happy so the AI wouldn't kill them for being an error in the system.

With all this hyper-surveillance culture we risk creating a society where rest is no longer a sanctuary, but a site of extraction. The bedroom becomes another factory floor, where we are generating data for brokers and proving our worth to employers. To truly own the night means reclaiming the right to sleep unobserved.

Legal Frameworks

We are currently living through a strange interregnum in legal history as our ability to extract biological data has vastly outpaced our ability to regulate it. We have 21st-century sensors operating under 20th-century laws. The average user operates under the assumption that their sleep data is classed as health data, and therefore protected by medical privacy laws. In most cases, this is a dangerous misconception. The legal status of your sleep depends entirely on who is collecting it.

In the United States, the primary shield for patient privacy is the Health Insurance Portability and Accountability Act (HIPAA). It is a robust law that makes it illegal for your doctor or hospital to share your medical records without your consent. However, HIPAA only applies to covered entities, i.e. healthcare providers, insurers, and clearinghouses. It does not apply to consumer technology companies. When you wear a Fitbit, an Oura ring, or an Apple Watch, you are not a patient; you are a user. The data you generate is not medical records; it is lifestyle data.

This distinction creates a massive regulatory wormhole known as the HIPAA gap. If a sleep lab measures your sleep apnoea, that data is locked down. If a gadget you bought at Best Buy measures the exact same apnoea events, that data is commercially tradable (subject only to the company's own privacy policy and state-level consumer protection laws). You effectively waive your medical privacy the moment you agree to the Terms of Service.

Europe has taken a different approach. The General Data Protection Regulation (GDPR) does not care if the data comes from a doctor or a watch; it cares about the nature of the data itself. Under Article 9 of the GDPR, health data is classified as 'Special Category Data'. This is the nuclear option of privacy law. Processing it requires explicit consent, which is a much higher bar than the standard 'I agree' tick-box exercise. It bans the processing of biometric data for the purpose of uniquely identifying a natural person unless strict exceptions are met. Crucially, the GDPR grants citizens the right to erasure (the right to be forgotten) and data portability. This means a European user can legally demand that a sleep tracker company delete every millisecond of data they ever collected, or export it in a readable format to take to a competitor. For the American user, these rights are a patchwork of state laws (like the CCPA in California), often leaving them with no delete button *per se* for their own biology.

While data privacy laws protect the record of sleep, a new class of labour laws is emerging to protect the act of sleep. These are the 'Right to Disconnect' laws. Originating in France (*le droit à la déconnexion*), and now adopted in varying forms by countries like Belgium, Portugal, and Australia, these laws recognise that the smartphone has dissolved the physical boundary of the factory. They provide a legal shield for the employee who refuses to answer emails or Slack messages outside of contracted hours. In Portugal, for example, it is illegal for employers to contact staff outside of work hours except in emergencies. In Belgium, federal civil servants have a statutory right to turn off their devices. These are not just labour laws; they are public health interventions. They are the first legislative attempts to ring-fence the biological night from the economic day. They establish the legal principle that your neurochemistry is not company property.

The next frontier of regulation is the Artificial Intelligence Act, recently passed by the EU. This legislation targets the inference engines we discussed in the previous section. The AI Act classifies AI systems used in critical infrastructure and essential private and public services as High Risk. Crucially, it creates strict guardrails for emotion recognition systems in the workplace. If a trucking company wants to use a AI camera to monitor a driver's eyelids for fatigue, or if a hedge fund wants to use sleep data to predict a trader's burnout risk, they will face rigorous scrutiny regarding accuracy, transparency, and human oversight. This combats the 'black box' problem and nudges us towards the 'glass box'. It forces companies to prove that their sleep algorithms are not just snake oil, and more importantly, that they are not being used to discriminate against workers based on invisible biological traits.

Looking further ahead, legal scholars are beginning to advocate for a new category of human rights: 'Neuro-Rights'. Spearheaded by legal ethicists and already finding its way into the constitution of Chile, this framework argues that the brain (and its states of consciousness, including sleep) requires specific constitutional protection.

It proposes the 'Right to Mental Privacy' which is the absolute right to keep your neural data (brainwaves, dreams, cognitive state) private. As sleep tech moves from the wrist (movement) to the head (EEG headbands and dream incubation), this will become the critical battleground. If a device can read your dreams or insert ads into your hypnagogic state, it is no longer a data privacy issue; it is a cognitive liberty issue. The legal frameworks are slowly waking up to the reality of the programmable night. But for now, the user remains the sheriff of their own data. Until the laws close the HIPAA gap and globalise the right to disconnect, 'owning the night' remains a personal responsibility rather than a guaranteed right.

Interoperability

If you are a typical quantified self-enthusiast, your biological life is currently fragmented across a dozen different servers. Your heart rate data lives in the Apple cloud. Your sleep stages live on Oura's servers in Finland. Your nutrition logs are in MyFitnessPal, owned by a private equity firm. Your genetic risk factors are sitting in 23andMe's new owner's database. These datasets describe the same organism, *you*, but they do not speak the same language. They are trapped in data silos. This fragmentation is not a technical accident; it is a deliberate business strategy known as the walled garden. In the tech industry, data is gravity. Companies know that the more historical data they hold on you, the harder it is for you to leave. If you have five years of sleep trends stored in the Fitbit ecosystem, switching to an Apple Watch feels like a lobotomy. You lose your history and you start from zero, which feels like a massive loss rather than a restart. This lock-in ensures brand loyalty not through superior innovation, but through the threat of data amnesia.

The cost of this fragmentation across apps and devices is high. It prevents us from seeing the holistic picture of our health. Sleep does not happen in a vacuum. It is deeply interconnected with what you ate for dinner (nutrition app), how much you moved (fitness app), the temperature of your bedroom (smart thermostat), and your stress levels (meditation app). To truly engineer sleep, we need to be able to overlay these graphs. We need to be able to ask complex questions like: *Does my deep sleep suffer on days when I run more than 5km and eat dairy* Or, *Does the humidity in my bedroom correlate with my wake-ups?*

Currently, answering these questions requires a spreadsheet and hours of manual data entry. The interoperability movement seeks to automate this. It fights for a world where your biological data is fluid, portable, and platform-agnostic. The technical solution to this problem already exists. It is an unsexy but revolutionary standard called Fast Healthcare Interoperability Resources (FHIR). Developed by the healthcare industry to allow hospitals to talk to each other, FHIR is essentially a universal translator for the body. It defines how a heart rate or a sleep session should be coded so that any computer system can understand it. Effectively it is a unifier of metadata and sensors.

We are seeing a push to force consumer wearables to adopt this standard. If Oura, Apple, and Whoop all output their data in FHIR format, you could theoretically plug them all into a neutral biological dashboard app. You could then swap hardware as easily as you swap a lightbulb, without losing your data history (one is not available at the time of writing).

Imagine a Health OS that sits above the brands. You wake up and look at a single screen.

- **Layer 1:** It pulls your sleep data from your ring.
- **Layer 2:** It pulls the CO_2 levels and temperature from your Netatmo weather station.
- **Layer 3:** It pulls your calendar data (stress load) from Google.
- **Layer 4:** It pulls your spending data (late-night Uber Eats) from your bank or payment app.

The system then runs a cross-correlation analysis. It tells you: *You sleep 15% deeper when the room is below 19°C and you haven't spent money on food after 8pm.* This is the promise of interoperability. It turns isolated metrics into actionable wisdom. Whether you follow that wisdom to make improvements to your life is still your choice.

Until that future arrives, the user's primary weapon is the data export function.

Under GDPR in Europe and CCPA in California, almost every tech company is legally required to provide a button that says 'Download My Data'. However, companies often engage in malicious compliance. They will let you download your data, but they will give it to you in a PDF format. A PDF is dead data. You can read it, but a computer cannot easily process it, it is a digital piece of paper. True interoperability requires machine-readable formats like JSON or CSV. These are the live files that can be imported into other systems. When you are choosing a sleep tracker, you should always check their export policy. If they only give you a PDF, they are trying to lock you in. If they give you a CSV/JSON, they respect your ownership.

The endgame of interoperability is a concept called the Personal Data Store (or Solid Pod, a project led by Sir Tim Berners-Lee, inventor of the Web). In this model, your data does not live on Apple's servers or Google's servers. It lives in a secure pod that *you* own. You grant apps permission to visit your data, but they cannot take it with them.

- You download a sleep analysis app. It asks: 'Can I read your sleep logs for the last month?'
- You say 'Yes'.
- The app comes into your pod, analyses the numbers, gives you a report, and then leaves.
- If you delete the app, the data stays with you. The app leaves with nothing.

This reverses the current power dynamic. Currently, the app owns the data and rents it back to you. In the PDS model, you own the land, and the apps are just visitors.

Interoperability is not just a technical specification; it is a freedom. It is the right to pick up your biological history and walk away. It forces companies to compete on the quality of their insights, not the height of their walls. As we move into a future where our health is increasingly digitised, we must demand that our data remains fluid. We must reject the walled gardens that try to turn our bodies into proprietary platforms. Your sleep belongs to you, and you should be able to take it wherever you go.

The Future of Data Rights

We stand at a crossroads in the history of human identity. For millennia, the definition of self was philosophical and physical. It was your thoughts, your actions, and the body you inhabited. But in the 21st century, the self has expanded into the digital realm. It now includes a digital exhaust plume of terabytes; the record of every heartbeat, every REM cycle, every cortisol spike, and every genetic risk factor.

Currently, we exist in a state of data feudalism, we are the serfs working the land. We generate the raw material (the biological data) through the labour of living and sleeping. But we do not own the land. The landlords, aka the tech giants and data aggregators, own the servers, the algorithms, and ultimately, the value derived from our bodies. They grant us the privilege of seeing our own data on a dashboard, but they retain the power to sell it, mine it, or lock us out of it. The future of data rights demands a revolution. It demands the overthrow of this feudal model and its replacement with a model of biological sovereignty.

In law, *Habeas Corpus* (that you have the body) is the fundamental right that protects against unlawful imprisonment. We need a digital equivalent: Data *Habeas Corpus*.

This principle asserts that your biological data is not a commodity you create; it is an extension of your physical person. Therefore, it cannot be sold, seized, or exploited without your explicit, revocable, and granular consent. Under this framework, a Terms of Service agreement that claims perpetual ownership of your sleep data would be unconstitutional. You cannot sign away your human rights, and you should not be able to sign away your neural rights.

The technological architecture for this future is already being built. It is called Self-Sovereign Identity (SSI). In the current web (Web 2.0), your identity consists of rented profiles: you log in with Google, or you log in with Facebook. If they ban you, you disappear.

In an SSI model (Web 3.0), your identity is a cryptographic key that *you* hold. Your sleep data is attached to this key. It sits in your digital wallet, encrypted.

- When you visit a doctor, you use your key to grant them temporary access to your sleep history.
- When you join a new gym, you grant them read-only access to your recovery scores.
- When you stop paying the gym, you turn the key, and their access instantly vanishes.

This shifts the power dynamic from 'please delete my data' (a request they might ignore) to 'I have revoked your access (a mathematical certainty).

One individual fighting Google is a losing battle. But ten million individuals is a union. We are seeing the emergence of data 'Trusts' or data 'Unions'. Imagine a union for sleeping humans: Millions of users pool their sleep data into a secure, democratically governed trust; some might also call this a Decentralised, Autonomous Organisation (DAO) in Web 3.0.

- If a pharmaceutical company wants to train an AI to detect insomnia using this dataset, they cannot just scrape it for free. They must negotiate with the Union.
- The Union demands a fee. That fee is then redistributed as a data dividend to the users.
- The Union also sets ethical standards. They might say, 'We will not sell data to insurance companies or political campaigns'.

This treats data not as waste to be harvested, but as capital to be invested. It acknowledges that the trillion-dollar AI industry is built on *our* data, and we deserve a seat at the table, and a share of the cheque.

As discussed in previous sections, the biggest danger is not what you share, but what the AI guesses. The future of data rights must include protection against non-consensual inference. It should be illegal to infer a health condition (like pregnancy, dementia, or depression) from non-health data (like shopping habits or sleep timing) without consent. You have a right to your secrets. If an algorithm figures out you are sick before you tell your doctor, that algorithm has violated your privacy just as surely as a peeping tom.

Finally, we must demand a shift in software architecture towards 'Zero-Knowledge Proofs'. This is a cryptographic method where a system can verify a fact about you without seeing the raw data. For example, an insurance company needs to know: *Does this person sleep enough to qualify for the low-risk discount?*

- **Current Model:** You send them your entire sleep log. They see everything including your late nights, your insomnia, your intimacy.
- **Zero-Knowledge Model:** Your phone runs a calculation locally. It generates a cryptographic proof that says: *Yes, this user averages >7 hours.* It sends *only* that Y token to the insurer. The insurer gets the verification they need; you keep your privacy.

We (the GenX and Millennials) are the first generations in history to be fully quantified. We are the test subjects. The precedents we set now in the courts, in the code, and in our culture, will define human privacy for the next century.

To 'own the night' is to reject the idea that we are merely content generators for the cloud. It is to assert that our dreams, our rhythms, and our biology are sovereign territory. The technology to protect us exists; we just need the political will to demand it. We must ensure that as we drift off to sleep, we are not logging in to a surveillance state, but resting securely within a sanctuary of our own making. It's really not too much to ask.

10

Motherhood and Menopause

> For decades, women have been treated as 'small men' in medical research.
>
> But a woman's sleep architecture is fundamentally different. We are not just smaller; we are cyclical.
>
> DR. ALYSON MCGREGOR

The Gender Data Gap

For the majority of modern medical history, the 'standard' human was a 70-kilogram white male. He was the baseline for drug dosages, the crash test dummy for car safety, and the reference point for understanding human physiology. Women were viewed not as a distinct biological category, but as small men with hormones.

This bias is particularly acute in sleep science. For decades, researchers actively excluded women from sleep studies. The reasoning was, ironically, the very thing that made studying women so necessary: hormonal variability. The menstrual cycle, with its fluctuating levels of estrogen and progesterone, introduced 'noise' into the clean datasets researchers craved. So, they studied men, assuming the results would map perfectly onto women.

They do not. The exclusion of female physiology has created a profound *Gender Data Gap* in our understanding of the night. It has led to diagnostic criteria that miss female-specific sleep disorders and to technology that is fundamentally miscalibrated for half the population.

The Biological Blind Spot

The male sleep cycle is relatively static. It follows a 24-hour circadian rhythm. The female sleep cycle involves a second, infradian rhythm, aka the menstrual cycle, which overlays the circadian one. During the follicular phase (after menstruation), a woman's sleep architecture might resemble the male baseline. But during the luteal phase (the second half of the cycle), progesterone spikes. This hormone is a potent soporific; it acts on GABA receptors similarly to Valium, however, it also raises core body temperature by roughly 0.5 degrees Celsius.

As we discussed earlier in Chapter 4, a drop in core body temperature is the trigger for sleep onset and deep sleep. When the biological baseline is raised during the luteal phase, the body has to work harder to cool down. This fight against internal heat leads to fragmented sleep, vivid dreams, and a reduction in REM. For decades, women reporting this cyclical exhaustion were dismissed as anxious or moody. The science didn't validate their experience because the science hadn't measured it.

This historical bias has been hard-coded into the first generation of sleep technology. The algorithms that power the world's most popular smartwatches and rings were largely trained on male-skewed datasets. Consider the 'Readiness Score': These scores often penalise a user for an elevated resting heart rate or a slightly higher body temperature. For a man, these metrics usually signal stress, illness, or overtraining. For a woman, they might simply signal ovulation or the luteal phase.

A woman in the second half of her cycle might wake up feeling fine, but her device tells her she is unrecovered because her temperature is up. The device is gaslighting her biology. It is interpreting a healthy hormonal fluctuation as a pathological error. This not only renders the data useless; it creates unnecessary anxiety by telling women they are failing at sleep when they are simply functioning as women.

The gap extends to medical diagnosis. Obstructive Sleep Apnoea (OSA) has traditionally been viewed as a male disease:

the overweight man snoring loudly. Women with OSA present differently. They are less likely to snore loudly and more likely to report insomnia, morning headaches, and fatigue. Because these symptoms don't fit the male checklist, women are frequently misdiagnosed with depression and prescribed antidepressants, which can actually worsen sleep quality.

We are finally seeing a correction and are seeing the rise of menstrual-aware algorithms where newer wearable platforms are beginning to ask users to log their cycle. They are adjusting their baselines dynamically e.g. recognising that a higher temperature in week three is normal, not fever. They are beginning to map the distinct sleep architecture of the female brain, which tends to have more robust slow wave sleep but greater vulnerability to arousal.

Closing the gender data gap is not just about fairness; it is about precision engineering. We cannot build a 'Programmable Sanctuary' for a woman using the blueprints designed for a man. To own the night, we must first acknowledge that the female night is biologically distinct, governed by a different clock, and deserving of its own science.

Pregnancy and Postpartum

If the gender data gap is an oversight, the treatment of sleep during pregnancy and the postpartum period is a crisis. For generations, the medical establishment has shrugged at the exhaustion of new mothers. *You're pregnant; you're supposed to be tired*, or *You have a newborn; you won't sleep*. These platitudes dismiss what is, largely, a solvable physiological engineering problem. Pregnancy is a supreme stress test for the body. It involves massive hormonal shifts, biomechanical restructuring, and hemodynamic changes. In the first trimester, soaring progesterone acts as a heavy sedative, yet sleep is often unrefreshing. By the third trimester, physical discomfort e.g. back pain, bladder pressure, and restless legs syndrome (which affects up to 30 per cent of pregnant women), makes continuous sleep nearly impossible.

Then comes the fourth trimester aka the newborn phase aka my brain in a jar phase. Here, the challenge shifts from internal biology to external interruption. The sleep deprivation of a new parent is a very specific form of torture: fragmentation. It is not just the lack of hours; it is the inability to complete a full sleep cycle. This fragmentation destroys executive function and emotional regulation, leading to the dangerous fog of postpartum depression and anxiety. Both of whom I have been personally acquainted to despite me not wanting to know them.

The primary challenge in treating pregnancy insomnia is safety. Standard pharmacological interventions such as sedatives and hypnotics, are generally contraindicated or used with extreme caution due to potential risks to the foetus. This leaves the pregnant woman with few options. Enter Digital Cognitive Behavioural Therapy for Insomnia (dCBTI). This is the 'software as a drug' revolution. Apps like Sleepio (developed at Harvard) or Somryst (only available in the USA with medical supervision/prescription) use algorithms to deliver the gold-standard psychological treatment for insomnia without a single chemical molecule.

CBTI works by restructuring the cognitive associations with the bed and using Sleep Restriction Therapy (SRT) to build high sleep pressure. In a clinical setting, this is expensive and hard to access. As an app, it is scalable and available at 3am. For pregnant women, dCBTI offers a lifeline. It provides a way to manage the insomnia of anxiety; the racing thoughts about the birth or parenthood, using proven cognitive techniques, with zero risk to the developing baby.

Once the baby arrives, the engineering goal shifts. The fourth trimester theory posits that human infants are born three months early compared to other mammals, due to our large brain size of the baby and relative pelvic size of the mother. They are not ready for the cold, still, silent world. They crave the environment of the womb: constant motion and constant noise (the shushing of blood flow). This is the logic behind the smart bassinet where devices like the Snoo are essentially robotic uteruses. They use microphones to detect when the baby is crying and respond automatically. They escalate the intensity of rocking and white noise to soothe the infant back to sleep. Critics call them lazy parenting. Engineers call them responsive loop systems. They do not replace feeding or changing; they replace the 45 minutes of rocking required to settle a fussy baby. By adding one or two hours of sleep to the baby's night, they add one or two hours to the parents' night. In the context of postpartum mental health, those two hours are not a luxury; they are a medical necessity.

We have also seen the rise of smart socks and computer vision cameras (like the Owlet or Nanit). These devices track the infant's heart rate and oxygen saturation (Pulse Oximetry) or monitor the rise and fall of their chest. For parents of premature babies or those with medical anxieties, this data is a godsend. It offers peace of mind, however, as discussed in the Orthosomnia section, it can backfire on your plans for more rest and peace. If the parameters are set too sensitively, the device generates false alarms. A parent who is woken up at 2am by a blaring siren because the sock slipped off a kicking foot suffers a massive cortisol spike. Instead of sleeping when the baby sleeps, the parent lies awake, staring at the app, watching the green line of the heart rate.

The advice here is selective deployment i.e. use the technology to prevent tragedy, but do not use it to micromanage the night. If the baby is healthy and full-term, constant biometric surveillance may cause more anxiety than it cures.

The final piece of the puzzle is light. A newborn has no circadian rhythm. Their pineal gland does not produce melatonin for the first few months. They operate on ultradian cycles of hunger and digestion. They are essentially jet-lagged time travellers. The parents' job is to act as the external circadian clock. This requires rigorous light engineering in the nursery.

- **Daytime:** Exposure to bright, natural daylight is crucial. It signals wakefulness to the infant's developing brain.

- **The Night Feed:** This is the critical failure point. When a baby cries at 3am, many parents turn on a lamp or check their phones. This blasts both the parent and the baby with blue-enriched light, suppressing melatonin and waking everyone up fully.

The programmable sanctuary for a new parent *must* rely on red light. Red light (long wavelength) does not trigger the ipRGCs (those pesky light sensing retinal cells) in the eye. It allows you to see the diaper and the bottle without signalling 'morning' to the brain. A nursery equipped with motion-activated, dim red LEDs allows for the stealth feed; in, change, feed, out, without breaking the biological night.

Technology cannot remove the burden of parenthood. The baby will still wake up. But by using dCBTI to protect maternal sleep quality, smart bassinets to extend infant sleep duration, and red light to protect circadian alignment, we can turn a period of exhaustion into a period of manageable fatigue. We can engineer a softer landing for the new family, especially the ones who can afford all the equipment.

The Menopausal Transition

If adolescence is the construction site of the brain, the menopausal transition is its renovation. It is a period of profound neurobiological rewiring, yet in the sleep clinic or during the design of wearables, it is often treated with a shrug or not even considered. A woman presents with sudden, intractable insomnia in her late forties. She is often told it is 'just aging' or 'stress', but in reality, she is experiencing a specific, chaotic failure of her internal climate control system.

The primary saboteur of sleep during perimenopause and menopause is the Vasomotor Symptom (VMS), colloquially known as the hot flash or night sweat. While these are often played for laughs in popular culture, biologically, they are violent events. They represent a momentary collapse of the body's ability to thermoregulate. Deep in the brain lies the hypothalamus. Among its many jobs, it acts as the body's thermostat, maintaining our core temperature within a tight thermoneutral zone. Estrogen plays a critical role in stabilising this zone. As estrogen levels fluctuate and eventually plummet during the menopausal transition, this zone narrows significantly. The thermostat becomes hypersensitive.

A tiny fluctuation in ambient temperature or a minor internal shift that would normally be ignored triggers a massive overheating alarm. The hypothalamus panics. It thinks the body is burning up. In a desperate attempt to dump heat, it dilates the blood vessels in the skin (vasodilation) and triggers the sweat glands.

For the sleeper, this is a catastrophic interruption. The sequence usually looks like this:

1. **The Surge:** A surge of adrenaline and norepinephrine hits the system.
2. **The Heat:** Intense heat floods the chest and face.

3. **The Wake-Up:** The brain is jolted out of deep sleep into full wakefulness. This is not a gentle rising; it is a chemical emergency.
4. **The Chill:** The sweat evaporates, and because the body wasn't actually overheating to begin with, the core temperature plummets. The sleeper is now freezing, shivering in damp sheets.

This cycle can happen once a night or twenty times a night. It shreds sleep architecture. Even if the woman does not fully wake up (a micro-arousal), the brain is pulled out of restorative Slow Wave Sleep into lighter stages to manage the thermal crisis. She wakes up exhausted, not realising she has run a neurological marathon all night.

The impact extends beyond the thermal event itself. The unpredictability of these attacks creates a secondary layer of anticipatory anxiety. The bed becomes a site of potential ambush. This hyperarousal makes it difficult to fall back asleep after an attack, leading to maintenance insomnia. Furthermore, the loss of estrogen and progesterone has direct effects on sleep centres independent of temperature. Progesterone is a natural respiratory stimulant; as it drops, the airway becomes more collapsible. This is why the risk of Obstructive Sleep Apnoea (OSA) skyrockets in post-menopausal women, often equalling the risk in men, yet women are rarely screened for it.

Understanding the menopausal transition requires reframing it. It is not a psychological issue of mid-life crisis; it is a physiological issue of neurological withdrawal. The brain is learning to function without the neuro-protective and sleep-promoting hormones (estrogen/progesterone) it has relied on for thirty years. It is a turbulent recalibration. Recognising this and naming the hot flash not as a nuisance but as a specific disruptor of the sleep cycle, is the first step toward managing it. We cannot simply relax our way through a broken thermostat; we have to engineer a solution.

Tech for Thermal Relief

If the menopausal hot flash is a failure of the body's internal climate control, then the solution is external engineering. For decades, the advice given to women was analog and patronising; dress in layers, keep a fan by the bed, or open a window. These are passive strategies. They deal with the heat after it has already woken you up.

The new wave of thermal technology is active. It moves beyond simple cooling to autonomic modulation and predictive intervention. The goal is not just to cool the skin, but to trick the brain into believing it is cool, thereby aborting the hot flash before it reaches the catastrophic wake-up phase.

The most elegant breakthrough in this space comes from understanding the biology of the wrist. The inside of the wrist is highly innervated with thermoreceptors that have a direct hotline to the hypothalamus; the brain's thermostat. This biological loophole has given rise to devices like the Embr Wave. It looks like a smartwatch, but it is actually a high-precision

Peltier plate (a thermoelectric heat pump). When a woman feels the prodrome i.e. subtle, rising anxiety or warmth that precedes a hot flash by about thirty seconds; she taps the device. It immediately delivers a focused, intense wave of cold to the inner wrist. This sensation does not physically cool the entire body; the device is too small for that. Instead, it sends a thermal rescue signal to the brain. The intense local cold tells the hypothalamus: *We are interacting with something cold. Stand down.* This interrupts the panic signal. It can stop the vasodilation and sweating response in its tracks. It is hacking the sensation of temperature to control the reality of temperature.

Research has shown that this pulsed thermal sensation is more effective than constant cooling. If you hold an ice cube, your nerves go numb and stop reporting the cold. By pulsing the temperature in waves, the device keeps the nerves alert and the signal to the brain active. It provides relief without the discomfort of freezing the skin.

While wrist wearables are excellent for the daytime, they require the user to be awake enough to press a button. At night, the goal is to never wake up at all. This requires automation. We are seeing the emergence of closed-loop cooling mattresses designed specifically for menopause. Systems like the Terra by Amira or advanced configurations of the Eight Sleep Pod represent a leap forward. These are not just water-cooled pads; they are predictive engines. These systems use biometric sensors to monitor heart rate variability (HRV) and movement in real-time. A hot flash is rarely silent; it is often preceded by a distinct spike in heart rate and a drop in HRV as the sympathetic nervous system kicks in.

The AI in these mattress covers learns this signature. When it detects the physiological ramp-up of a flash, it triggers a rapid cooling response *before* the user wakes up. It pumps chilled water through the pad, effectively dumping the excess body heat into the mattress. The concept is thermal interception. By neutralising the heat spike instantly, the system prevents the micro-arousal that fragments sleep. The user might still have the flash, but they sleep through it. They wake up dry, rather than drenched, because the sweat response was rendered unnecessary by the external cooling.

Between the body and the bed lies the fabric. Traditional cotton or silk can become saturated with sweat, turning cold and clammy; a phenomenon known as the post-flash chill. This chill is often what wakes women up, rather than the heat itself.

The solution lies in Phase Change Materials (PCMs). Originally developed by NASA to protect astronauts from extreme temperature fluctuations, these materials are now being woven into menopause-grade pyjamas and sheets. PCMs work on a molecular level. They contain microscopic capsules of paraffin or bio-based wax. When the body heats up, the wax inside the capsule melts, absorbing the thermal energy and pulling heat away from the skin. When the body cools down (during the post-flash chill), the wax solidifies, releasing the stored heat back to the skin. This creates a thermal buffer.

It flattens the curve of temperature fluctuation. Instead of a sharp spike and a sharp drop, the sleeper experiences a gentle wave. Brands like Dagsmejan or Femography use these fabrics to create a dry zone around the skin, preventing the clamminess that disrupts sleep continuity.

The holy grail of this technology is complete integration. Imagine a future where your wrist sensor detects the onset of a flash and wirelessly communicates with your HVAC system to blast cold air for ten minutes, while simultaneously telling your mattress to drop five degrees. This ecosystem approach acknowledges that menopause is a 24-hour condition that peaks at night. By combining autonomic modulation (the wrist), predictive active cooling (the bed), and passive buffering (the fabric), we can build a thermal fortress around the sleeper. We can turn the bedroom from a sweatbox into a responsive life-support system that handles the heat so the dreaming mind doesn't have to.

The Future of Women's Sleep Tech

For the first decade of the wearable revolution, the industry's approach to female physiology could be summarised by a marketing strategy known as 'pink it and shrink it'. Companies took devices designed for male biology, painted them rose gold, made the strap smaller, and perhaps added a manual period tracker that functioned little better than a paper calendar. This was not engineering; it was cosmetic pandering. As we look to the future, we are seeing the emergence of a new paradigm: *Femtech 2.0*. This is not about aesthetic adaptation;

it is about physiological-first design. It acknowledges that a woman's sleep is not just a circadian event, but a complex interplay of circadian and infradian (cycle-long) rhythms. The future of sleep technology for women moves beyond tracking to dynamic interpretation and diagnostic equity.

The most critical software update required for the female sleeper is the Dynamic Baseline. Currently, most algorithms use a static baseline. They calculate your normal heart rate and temperature based on a 30-day average. If you deviate from this average, the device assumes something is wrong. But a woman *should* deviate from those so-called norms. As we discussed, during the luteal phase, her resting heart rate rises and her HRV drops. A static algorithm sees this as stress or poor recovery and advises her to rest, often leading to frustration or anxiety.

Future algorithms; already in beta testing with forward-thinking companies like Oura and Whoop, will be cycle-aware. They will know that in Week 3, a higher temperature is not a fever; it is progesterone. They will adjust the 'Readiness Score' expectation accordingly.

- **The Follicular Mode:** The device might say: *Your physiology is primed for high intensity. Push hard today.*
- **The Luteal Mode:** The device might switch: *Your body is prioritising endometrial maintenance. Your baseline recovery is lower. Aim for stability, not peak performance.*

This shifts the relationship from judgment to validation. The device stops gaslighting the user and starts supporting her biological reality.

The next frontier is using sleep data to diagnose invisible female diseases. Conditions like Polycystic Ovary Syndrome (PCOS) and Endometriosis take an average of seven to ten years to diagnose. Yet, both conditions leave distinct fingerprints on sleep architecture long before they are clinically confirmed.

- **PCOS:** Often correlated with a specific signature of sleep fragmentation and a higher risk of sleep apnoea even in non-obese women.
- **Endometriosis:** Linked to pain-induced micro-arousals; tiny spikes in heart rate during the night that do not fully wake the sleeper but prevent deep sleep consolidation.

Future sleep trackers will act as an early warning system. By analysing the *texture* of the night, not just the duration, AI models will be able to flag these patterns. A notification might read: *We've noticed a cyclical pattern of micro-arousals that correlates with your reported cycle. This sleep signature is consistent with endometriosis. Consider sharing this report with your gynaecologist.* This turns the sleep tracker into a reproductive health tool.

As Hormone Replacement Therapy (HRT) becomes de-stigmatised and more widely prescribed for menopausal symptom management, tech will play a crucial role in dosage optimisation. Currently, HRT is often prescribed on a try and see basis. A woman takes a patch or a pill, and returns to the doctor in three months to report how she feels. This is slow and subjective. The 'Integrated Sleeper' of the future will link her medication log with her sleep data. The system could show: On the days you took your micronised progesterone at 7pm, your Deep Sleep increased by 15% compared to when you took it at 9pm. It turns the patient into an n=1 clinical trial, allowing for precise titration of hormones to maximise restorative sleep.

The End of the Standard Human

Ultimately, the future of women's sleep tech is about retiring the standard male model entirely. We are moving toward interoperable biological identity. We need devices that account for differences in skin thickness (which affects optical heart rate sensors), vascular density, and even the way sleep stages manifest in the female brain. We are moving toward a world where female is not a setting in a menu, but the default architecture of the device she wears. By closing the gender data gap, we do more than just sell more watches. We validate the experience of half the human species. We provide women with the tools to prove that their exhaustion is real, that their pain is visible in the data, and that their need for rest is not a weakness, but a biological imperative that deserves to be engineered with respect.

11

The Business of Dreams

> We are now in the age of the 'Sleep Economy'.
> We have taken a biological necessity and turned
> it into a lifestyle product.

FAST COMPANY / THE BUSINESS OF FASHION

Market Segmentation

For most of human history, sleep was not a commodity. It was a biological necessity, and largely free of commercial intervention. You bought a bed, perhaps a pillow, and that was the extent of the sleep economy. But in the twenty-first century, sleep has been transformed into one of the fastest-growing sectors of the global wellness market. It is now an industry worth hundreds of billions of dollars, driven by a simple, terrifying paradox: the more obsessed we become with sleep, the worse we seem to get at it, and the more we are willing to pay to fix it.

To understand this burgeoning behemoth, we cannot look at it as a single monolith. The sleep economy is a complex ecosystem composed of distinct, often competing segments. It is a war for the bedroom, fought on four primary fronts: Hardware, Pharmaceuticals, Environment (Mattresses/Bedding), and Services. Each of these segments targets a different aspect of the sleeper's anxiety, and each is evolving at a breakneck pace.

The most visible and disruptive segment is Sleep Technology, or #sleeptech. This is the domain of the sensor. It includes wearable trackers like the Apple Watch, Oura Ring, and Whoop strap, as well as nearables; devices that sit on the nightstand or under the mattress to monitor the sleeper without touching them. This segment is driven by the desire for data. It monetises our need for validation. The consumer in this segment is buying a mirror. They want to know, with metric precision, how well they rested. This market has exploded from a niche hobby for bio-hackers into a mainstream necessity.

As we have already discussed in this book: The hardware is increasingly sophisticated, moving from simple accelerometers (which just measure movement) to clinical-grade pulse oximeters and optical heart rate sensors that can detect atrial fibrillation or sleep apnoea. However, the hardware market is facing a saturation point. The wrist is crowded. This is driving a shift towards invisible hardware, e.g. smart rings, sensor-embedded sheets, and radar-based tracking that requires no compliance from the user. The goal is ambient intelligence: technology that disappears into the fabric of the room.

While the tech companies sell data, the pharmaceutical companies sell results. This is the oldest and most profitable segment of the sleep economy. It ranges from over-the-counter supplements like melatonin, magnesium, and valerian root to heavy-duty prescription hypnotics like Ambien. This market is currently undergoing a massive bifurcation. On one side, there is the wellness supplement boom. This is unregulated, brand-driven, and fuelled by social media trends. It sells the idea of natural sleep and targets the worried well; the people who sleep okay but want to sleep *perfectly*. On the other side is 'Big Pharma', which is pivoting away from the dangerous, addictive sedatives of the past (benzodiazepines) towards the new class of precision drugs like Dual Orexin Receptor Antagonists (DORAs). These drugs target the specific wakefulness pathways in the brain rather than just knocking the patient unconscious. This segment targets the clinically diagnosed insomniac, a population that is growing as the population ages and anxiety levels rise. The pharmaceutical promise is strikingly simple: *Swallow this, and the problem goes away.*

The third pillar is the sleep environment. This is the battle for the physical surface we sleep on. Historically, this was a sleepy industry dominated by a few legacy players who sold mattresses in confusing, fluorescent-lit showrooms. That model was detonated by the Bed-in-a-Box revolution. Direct-to-consumer (DTC) brands like Casper, Purple, and Simba used venture capital to bypass the showroom, shipping compressed foam mattresses directly to doorsteps with a 100-night trial. They turned a boring utility purchase into a lifestyle brand. But the foam wars have largely ended; the market is commoditised. The new frontier in this segment is active surfaces. We are seeing the merger of the mattress and the machine. Companies like Eight Sleep and Tempur-Pedic are releasing so-called smart beds that actively regulate temperature, adjust firmness in real-time based on your sleeping position, and vibrate to wake you up without an alarm. The mattress is no longer just a cushion; it is a personalised sleep-butler robot selling optimisation. It targets the high-performer who views their bed as a charging station for their biological battery.

The final, and perhaps most interesting, segment is 'Sleep Services'. Hardware gives you data; pills give you sedation; mattresses give you comfort. But none of them give you behaviour change. None of them fix the bad habits that are actually causing the insomnia; this gap is being filled by digital therapeutics and coaching platforms. This includes apps like Calm and Headspace (sleep stories and meditation), Sleepio (Digital Cognitive Behavioural Therapy for Insomnia), and high-end concierge coaching services where human experts analyse your data and tell you when to stop drinking coffee.

This industry segment is growing because we have realised that data alone is useless without context. Knowing you got 12 minutes of Deep Sleep is stressful; knowing *how* to increase it requires guidance. The services market is moving from content (listen to this rain sound) to therapy (follow this restriction protocol), and it is the software layer that sits on top of the hardware, trying to program the human into better hygiene. What makes the current moment so dynamic is that these boundaries are dissolving. The hardware companies are launching coaching services (Whoop). The mattress companies are building apps (Eight Sleep). The pharmaceutical companies are partnering with digital therapy apps (Somryst*).

We are seeing the formation of sleep ecosystems. Companies want to own the entire vertical; they don't just want to sell you a ring; they want to sell you the ring, the subscription to the app that analyses the ring data, the supplement recommended by the app, and the smart mattress that reacts to the ring's sensors. This segmentation reveals a fundamental truth about the modern condition: we have lost faith in our own ability to sleep and thereby we no longer trust our bodies to do the one thing they evolved to do perfectly. Instead, we are outsourcing the function to the market. We are building a scaffolding of products around our bed, hoping that if we buy enough sensors, swallow enough magnesium, and lie on enough cooling gel, we will finally find the rest that eludes us. The sleep economy is not just selling products; it is selling the promise of peace in a hyper-stimulated world. And as long as the world remains noisy, business will be good.

The Subscription Model

In the old economy, the transaction between a sleep company and a customer was simple and finite. You walked into a store, handed over cash for a mattress, a white noise machine, or a bottle of pills, and the relationship ended the moment you walked out the door. You owned the product, and the company had your money. If they wanted more of your money, they had to wait ten years for your mattress to sag or for your machine to break. This new transactional model is currently being systematically dismantled and replaced by the subscription economy. In the boardrooms of Silicon Valley and the strategy decks of major wellness brands, the holy grail is no longer the one-off sale; it is Annual Recurring Revenue (ARR). The goal is not to sell you a device; it is to turn you into a subscriber. The modern objective is to transform sleep from a product you buy into a service you rent.

The pioneer of this model in the wearable space was Whoop. When they launched, they did something radical: they didn't sell the strap. There was no upfront cost for the hardware. Instead, you paid a monthly membership fee (roughly US$30). As long as you paid, you got the strap, the upgrades, and the data. The moment you stopped paying, the device became a useless piece of fabric and plastic. This was a gamble, but it paid off. It shifted the psychological value from the *object* (the sensor) to the *insight* (the software). It acknowledged a fundamental truth of the tech industry: hardware is becoming commoditised. Accelerometers and heart rate sensors are cheap and anyone can build a tracker. The real value, aka the moat, is the proprietary algorithm that interprets that raw noise and tells you if you are ready to train or if you are about to get sick.

By charging for the membership, Whoop aligned its revenue model with its value proposition.

Other companies have followed suit, often clumsily. Oura, the maker of the smart ring, initially sold its device as a premium hardware purchase with no monthly fees. Users loved it. But with the launch of their Generation 3 ring, they introduced a mandatory monthly membership to access detailed sleep insights. The backlash was severe. Customers felt they were being held hostage as they had paid US$300 for a ring, but to see their own data, they had to pay a rent of US$6 a month. Despite the consumer friction, the economic logic is undeniable. Hardware companies live on a feast or famine cycle. They have a huge spike in revenue when a new device launches, followed by a long valley. Subscriptions smooth out this curve. They provide the steady cash flow required to fund the massive R&D teams that keep the algorithms accurate. For the company, a user who pays US$6 a month for five years is far more valuable than a user who buys a US$300 device once.

This model has given rise to the phenomenon of gated sleep quality. We are seeing a stratification of the sleeping experience based on your willingness to pay a monthly toll.

Consider the smart mattress sector. Eight Sleep, the leader in thermal regulation beds, sells a piece of hardware (the Pod cover) that costs over US$2,000. But to access the autopilot feature, aka the AI that automatically adjusts the temperature during the night based on your sleep stages, you must pay a subscription. Without the subscription, the US$2,000 smart cover becomes a dumb, manual electric blanket.

This creates a philosophical tension: Who owns the functionality of the device? If you buy a car, you don't expect to pay a monthly fee to use the air conditioning. But in the sleep economy, the air conditioning (the active cooling algorithm) is treated as a service, not a feature. The company argues that the algorithm is constantly learning and improving in the cloud, and therefore, you are paying for that ongoing intelligence. The consumer argues that they are paying a ransom to unlock hardware they have already purchased.

The danger of the subscription model is 'churn'; the rate at which customers cancel. In a transactional model, the company doesn't care if you stop using the treadmill after a month; they already have your money. In a subscription model, if you stop using the device, you stop paying. This puts immense pressure on sleep tech companies to prove their value every single month. They cannot just let you sleep; they have to *engage* you. This drives the gamification and content strategies we see exploding across the sector.

It is no longer enough for an app to just track your sleep, it must now offer you sleep Journalism (daily reports), coaching (AI chatbots giving advice), and content libraries (meditations, soundscapes, stretching videos). The app must become a destination and this is why we see hardware companies pivoting to become media companies. They are terrified that you will get bored of the data. Once you know your average sleep score is 85, why keep paying? To prevent you from leaving, they have to constantly invent new metrics (Stress Monitor, Resilience Score, Chronotype Analysis) to reignite your curiosity.

There is a deeper, more insidious implication of this model: the tenant relationship with your own biology. When you subscribe to a sleep service, your data lives on their servers. If you cancel your membership, you essentially lose access to your longitudinal history. You might be able to export a raw CSV file, but the beautiful graphs, the trends, and the actionable insights vanish. This creates a lock-in effect that is far more powerful than brand loyalty. You cannot leave because you cannot take your digital sleep identity with you. You are renting access to your own physiological history, this makes the switching cost incredibly high. If you have three years of data in the Fitbit ecosystem, then switching to Apple means erasing your memory. You are starting from zero. This 'data gravity' ensures that once a user enters a subscription ecosystem, they rarely leave, effectively guaranteeing the company a lifetime revenue stream.

As subscription fatigue sets in and to cost of living starts to bite, consumers are already paying for Netflix, Spotify, Amazon Prime, and cloud storage, the sleep economy will likely move towards the 'Great Bundle' or 'one ring to rule them all' approach. We are already seeing this with Apple One. You pay one fee for Music, TV, Cloud, and Fitness+. It is inevitable that Health+ will be added, bundling advanced sleep tracking into the ecosystem. Independent sleep companies will struggle to compete with these mega-bundles (be acquired or file for bankruptcy).

We may also see the rise of 'Sleep-as-a-Service' (SaaS) in the physical realm. Imagine a model where you do not buy a mattress at all, just pay US$100 a month. Company XYZ installs a state-of-the-art smart bed in your home. Every two years, they come and upgrade the hardware to the newest sensor model. If the cooling pump breaks, they replace it instantly. It is the iPhone Upgrade Program applied to the bedroom. In this future, you own nothing. You lease your comfort. You rent your temperature. And your ability to get a good night's sleep becomes a line item on your credit card statement, right next to your electricity bill. The business of sleep is betting that you will pay for it, because the alternative (untracked, unoptimised, analog unconsciousness) has been successfully rebranded as a failure of performance. We are moving from a world where sleep was a free natural resource to a world where it is a premium utility, metered and billed by the month.

The Medical-Consumer Blur

For decades, there was an Iron Curtain separating the world of medical devices from the world of consumer gadgets. On one side stood the medical establishment. Their devices were beige, clunky, exorbitantly expensive, and rigorously tested. They lived in hospitals and clinics, guarded by doctors and regulated by strict government bodies like the FDA. On the other side stood the consumer electronics industry. Their devices were sleek, affordable, and designed for entertainment or general fitness. They lived in Apple Stores and Best Buys, and their data was legally regarded as for recreational purposes only.

Today, that curtain has been torn down. We are witnessing the rapid medicalisation of consumer tech and the simultaneous consumerisation of medical tech. The result is a messy, lucrative grey zone where a smartwatch is also a cardiologist, and a ring is also a sleep lab. This convergence is reshaping the business of healthcare, threatening the traditional gatekeepers of medicine, and creating a new, confusing reality for patients and doctors alike.

The pivotal moment in this shift occurred in 2018, when Apple announced the Series 4 Watch. It didn't just count steps or track calories; it featured an electrical heart sensor capable of taking an ECG right from the wrist. Crucially, Apple had obtained *De Novo* clearance from the FDA for its Atrial Fibrillation (AFib) detection algorithm. This was a watershed moment. A consumer tech giant had successfully navigated the regulatory labyrinth to put a Class II medical device on the wrists of millions of people who were not patients. It legitimised the wearable as a clinical tool.

Since then, the floodgates have opened. Samsung, Fitbit (now Google), Oura, and Withings have all rushed to add 'medical-grade' features to their lifestyle products. The latest battleground is sleep apnoea. Historically, diagnosing apnoea required a referral, a waitlist, and an expensive night in a hospital bed wired up like an astronaut (Polysomnography).

Now, the Apple Watch Series 10 and the Samsung Galaxy Watch can detect breathing disturbances and flag signs of moderate to severe sleep apnoea using nothing but an accelerometer.

This is a massive economic disruption. It effectively bypasses the primary care physician as the gatekeeper of diagnosis. The device screens the population at scale. The user gets a notification: *You might have sleep apnoea. Talk to your doctor.* The funnel for the sleep clinic has shifted from the doctor's office to the user's nightstand. However, this blur is fraught with semantic traps. Tech companies are masters of the regulatory dance. They often tout their devices as 'FDA Cleared', which sounds to the average consumer exactly like 'FDA Approved', but they are not the same thing. FDA approval is a rigorous process reserved for high-risk devices (like pacemakers) that requires proving safety and efficacy through massive clinical trials. 'FDA Clearance' (specifically the 510(k) pathway) is a lower bar. It simply requires the company to prove that their device is substantially equivalent to a device that is already on the market.

Tech companies tread a fine line, they want the marketing halo of medical accuracy to justify their subscription prices, but they desperately want to avoid the legal liability of being a medical provider. Their Terms of Service are explicit: *This device is not intended to diagnose, treat, or cure any disease.* Yet, the marketing implies exactly the opposite. They sell you a SpO2 sensor (medical language) but tell you it's for wellness monitoring (legal language). This creates a dangerous ambiguity where the user trusts the device as a doctor, but the company takes no responsibility when the device is wrong.

This convergence has created a crisis in the consultation room. Doctors are facing a data tsunami. Patients are arriving at appointments not just with symptoms, but with spreadsheets. They have six months of sleep staging data, heart rate variability graphs, and oxygen saturation trends exported from their ring. For the clinician, this is a nightmare. Firstly, they are not trained to interpret consumer-grade data, which often uses proprietary algorithms that are black boxes. Secondly, the data is often noisy and prone to artifacts and errors. Thirdly, and most importantly, the healthcare system is not built to bill for this. A doctor gets paid for the 15-minute visit; they do not get paid to spend an hour analysing a PDF from a Fitbit.

This leads to a potential clash of cultures. The 'Quantified Self' patient feels empowered and dismissed when the doctor ignores their data. The doctor feels overwhelmed and liable. *If the patient showed me the data, and I missed a signal in the noise, and they have a heart attack next week, do I get sued?* However, the smarter clinicians are beginning to adapt. We are seeing the rise of connected care platforms that act as middleware. These software layers ingest the raw data from Apple or Oura, filter out the noise, and present the doctor with a clean, clinically relevant dashboard. The future of medicine is not ignoring the wearable, but integrating it.

The final phase of this blur is the 'Digital Prescription'. We are moving toward a world where the doctor does not just prescribe a pill; they prescribe a device. In Germany, the DiGA (Digital Health Applications) act allows doctors to prescribe medical apps, and statutory health insurance *must* pay for them. In the US, we are seeing insurers subsidising Apple Watches or Oura Rings for members. The logic is purely economic: it is cheaper to buy a diabetic patient a US$300 watch to track their activity than to pay for a US$30,000 foot amputation caused by sedentary neglect.

This is where the sleep economy truly scales; when a sleep tracker transitions from a gadget you buy for Christmas to a therapeutic tool paid for by health insurance, the total addressable market explodes. Tech companies are currently hiring Chief Medical Officers and building clinical research teams not out of altruism, but because they want access to the trillion-dollar healthcare reimbursement firehose.

The risk of this blur is that we pathologise normal life's highs and lows. By putting a medical monitor on a healthy person, we risk turning them into a patient (with a patient mentality – what's wrong with me today?). A dip in deep sleep becomes a symptom and a momentary spike in heart rate becomes an event to be concerned about. We are creating a class of the worried well; people who are physically healthy but digitally sick, anxious about metrics that may not even be accurate.

Yet, the potential upside is undeniable. The old medical model was reactive, where we waited until you had a heart attack to treat you. The new consumer-medical model is proactive as it watches you 24/7/365. It catches the atrial fibrillation at 3am on a Tuesday while you are asleep. It notices the trend of declining HRV weeks before the burnout crash.

The wall is down. The tech companies are now healthcare companies, and the hospitals are becoming data centres. The winner in this new economy will be the company that can bridge the gap and turn the noise of the consumer night into the signal of medical truth.

Sleep Tourism

For the better part of a century, the hospitality industry operated on a simple, unspoken contract: they provided a bed, and you provided the exhaustion. A hotel room was, fundamentally, a storage unit for a human body in transit. The measure of a good hotel was cleanliness and perhaps a chocolate on the pillow. Sleep was assumed to be the natural byproduct of a comfortable mattress and heavy curtains. In the post-pandemic era, this passive model has been upended. We are witnessing the rise of *Sleep Tourism*, a travel trend that views the hotel not as a base for exploring a city, but as a clinic for repairing a mind. Travellers are no longer booking flights to see the Eiffel Tower or the Grand Canyon; they are booking flights to go unconscious. They are checking in to check out. The Instagram *new-mother* algorithm is full of women escaping their lives even for just 24 hours to sleep in a hotel bed (with the blackout blinds being of more interest than the room service meals).

The driving force behind this sector is the sleep deficit of the modern workforce. High-net-worth individuals are often the most sleep-deprived demographic. They are cash-rich but time-poor, living in a state of chronic jet lag and digital hyper-arousal. For this demographic, a good night's sleep has become the ultimate luxury good, scarcer than champagne and more valuable than a spa treatment. Hotels have responded by weaponising the bedroom. The *Sleep Suite* is the new *Presidential Suite*. These rooms are no longer defined by their square footage or their view, but by their biophilic design and technological isolation.

We see this in the hotel amenities arms race. It began innocently enough with pillow menus representing a choice between goose down, buckwheat, or memory foam. It has escalated into full-scale biological engineering. High-end brands like Six Senses and Equinox Hotels have partnered with sleep scientists to turn their rooms into circadian fortresses. Standard features now include hospital-grade soundproofing (sound transmission class ratings of 60+), circadian lighting systems that automatically shift from blue-enriched light in the morning to amber, melatonin-friendly light in the evening, and air purification systems that scrub the room of allergens and CO_2 to prevent stuffy room wake-ups. And how sad is it to think that I am so easily pleased when I see a Japanese toilet in the posh hotel bathroom.

The centrepiece of this new offering is the bed itself, it is the start of the smart bed tsunami. The era of the static spring mattress is ending in the luxury sector. It is being replaced by the active surface. Hotel chains are increasingly deploying smart beds from companies like Bryte and Eight Sleep. These are not merely comfortable; they are robotic. A guest at the Park Hyatt New York (from US$1500) can check into a *Restorative Sleep Suite* featuring a Bryte bed that uses AI to adjust the firmness of 100 different zones in real-time as the guest moves. It tracks their heart rate and respiration, and if it detects the guest waking up, it gently rocks them back to sleep with a subsonic oscillation. This integration allows for a portable sleep identity. In the future, you will not just check in with your passport; you will check in with your sleep profile. Imagine; the bed in Tokyo will automatically download your firmness preferences and temperature settings from the bed you slept in back in London. The hotel becomes a seamless extension of your home sanctuary. Sign me up, the amount of bad nights I have had in expensive hotels. If you know, you know.

Beyond the hardware lies the all-encompassing 'Sleep Retreat'. These are multi-day, immersive programs designed to rehabilitate the guest's relationship with rest. This is primary sleep tourism; where sleep is the sole purpose of the trip. At these retreats, the itinerary is inverted. Instead of waking up early for a hike, guests are encouraged to sleep in. The day is structured around down-regulation. You might start with a cryotherapy session to lower core body temperature, followed by a sleep yoga (Yoga Nidra) class to engage the parasympathetic nervous system. The sleep concierge is the new Sommelier. Instead of recommending a wine pairing, they recommend a sleep stack. They might prescribe a weighted blanket, a specific aromatherapy blend (e.g. lavender and bergamot), and a guided meditation track. Some properties offer clinical-grade diagnostics, strapping guests into polysomnography devices for a night to diagnose apnoea or restlessness, with a doctor reviewing the data over breakfast.

Why are hotels pivoting so aggressively to sleep? The answer is pure economics. The wealthy wellness traveller is a golden goose. Data from the Global Wellness Institute suggests that international wellness tourists spend 53% more than the average tourist. Domestic wellness tourists spend 178% per cent more. Sleep programs allow hotels to capture a greater share of the guest's wallet. A standard guest pays for the room and maybe a breakfast. A sleep tourist pays for the room, the 'Sleep Optimisation Package' ($200 premium), the massage ($250), the consultation with the sleep doctor ($500), and the retail upsell of the pyjamas and supplements ($300). Furthermore, it creates 'stickiness'. If a hotel cures your insomnia, you are loyal for life. You are not just a customer; you are a patient who has been healed. Brands like Hästens (the Swedish mattress maker) have launched their own 'Sleep Spa' hotels, effectively creating a 24-hour showroom where the guest pays to test-drive a US$50,000+ mattress.

There is, of course, a profound irony at the heart of sleep tourism. To access these sanctuaries of rest, guests often endure the most sleep-disruptive activity known to man: long-haul air travel. They fly across eight time zones, putting their circadian rhythms in a blender, in order to visit a retreat that promises to fix their circadian rhythms. This paradox is being addressed by the jet lag loop. Hotels are now partnering with apps like Timeshifter (used by astronauts) to begin the therapy before the guest even leaves home. The app tells the guest when to see light and when to avoid it three days before the flight. When they arrive, the hotel room lighting is pre-programmed to align with their target time zone, and their meals are timed to reset their internal liver clocks.

Sleep tourism represents the final frontier of the experience economy. We have monetised food (gastrotourism), we have monetised adventure (ecotourism), and now we have monetised silence. It signals a shift in societal values; rest is no longer seen as a lack of activity; it is seen as a peak performance activity. The ultimate status symbol is not the bag you carry or the car you drive; it is the quality of your deep sleep. And in the emerging sleep economy, the industry is betting that you will pay a premium to reclaim the peace that the modern world has stolen from you. The hotel of the future is not a place to stay; it is a machine for sleeping.

Investment Trends

If you want to know what the bedroom of 2030 will look like, you do not look at the patent filings of mattress companies; you look at the deal flow of Venture Capital (VC) firms. For years, sleep was considered a sleepy investment; a low-margin world of textiles and furniture. But in the last half-decade, the smart money has woken up. Sleep has been reclassified. It is no longer a sub-sector of 'Home Goods'; it is now a pillar of the longevity economy. This reclassification has opened the floodgates. Billions of dollars are flowing into the sector, but the direction of this river has shifted. Investors are no longer interested in funding another wrist tracker or a slightly fluffier pillow. They are placing their bets on three specific frontiers: The Invisible, The Clinical, and The Neural.

<u>Trend 1: The Death of the Wearable, The Rise of the Invisible</u>

The first major trend is a shift away from active compliance. Investors have realised that human beings are lazy. We do not want to charge a watch every day. We do not want to wear a bulky ring to bed. Friction kills data collection and quality. Consequently, capital is flowing toward nearables and ambient sensing. As we have discussed in this book, this is the technology that lives *in* the room, not *on* the body. We are seeing massive funding rounds for companies developing radar-based systems (like Google's Soli chip technology) that sit on a nightstand and track chest movements with millimetre-wave precision. We are seeing investment in smart surfaces; textiles embedded with piezoelectric sensors that can detect a heartbeat through a mattress topper.

The bet here is on Zero User Interface (Zero-UI). The future product is one you never touch. You simply lie down, and the room begins to measure you. This signals a future where sleep tracking is not a conscious choice, but a passive infrastructure, as invisible and omnipresent as Wi-Fi.

Trend 2: The Pivot to Clinical Validity

The wellness bubble has burst: The market is flooded with cheap trackers that offer sleep scores based on shaky science. Consumers are becoming sceptical, and investors are becoming discerning. The new gold standard for investment is FDA clearance. Venture capital is aggressively targeting companies that straddle the line between consumer tech and medical devices. They are funding startups that are not just building an app, but conducting double-blind randomised control trials to prove their efficacy. This is driving the rise of 'Digital Therapeutics' (DTx). Investors are pouring money into software platforms that treat insomnia (like Big Health's Sleepio) or sleep apnoea diagnostics (like Wesper). The goal is to build products that are reimbursable by health insurance. The business model shifts from selling a gadget to a consumer for US$100 to selling a therapy to an insurance company for US$1,000. For the consumer, this means the sleep tech of the future will likely be more expensive and harder to access without a prescription, but it will also be vastly more accurate.

Trend 3: Neuro-Modulation and The Closed Loop

Perhaps the most futuristic trend is the investment in 'Neuro-Modulation'. Investors are betting that tracking sleep is boring; controlling sleep is profitable. We are seeing a surge of interest in stimulation technologies. This includes companies building headbands that use Transcranial Alternating Current Stimulation (tACS) to electrically nudge the brain into deep sleep waves. It includes earbuds that use pink noise to entrain brain rhythms. It includes vagus nerve stimulators that physically vibrate the chest to force the parasympathetic nervous system to engage.

The holy grail investment here is the closed loop system. This is a device that reads the brainwaves in real-time (Input) and adjusts the stimulation in real-time (Output). For example, a headband that detects you are entering a nightmare and plays a specific tone to guide you into a lucid dream or a lighter sleep stage. This is the transition from 'Read-Only' sleep tech to 'Read-Write' sleep tech.

<u>Trend 4: The AI Sleep Agent</u>

Finally, there is the inevitable AI layer. Hardware is hard; software is scalable. VCs are heavily funding Generative AI models trained specifically on sleep data. The vision here is the 'Sleep Agent'. This is an AI that lives on your phone (or in your ear, or around your neck) and acts as a biological concierge. It doesn't just show you a graph; it ingests your calendar, your nutrition logs, and your ring data to give you hyper-personalised instructions. *You have a high-stress meeting at 8am tomorrow. Based on your recovery score, you should skip the morning gym session and sleep until 7:15am. I have already adjusted your alarm.* Investors are backing companies that can build these large action models: AIs that can take action in the real world (adjusting the thermostat, dimming the lights, cancelling an appointment) based on sleep data.

Conclusion: The Bifurcation of Sleep

What do these trends signal for the future availability of products? They signal a bifurcation of sleep. At the bottom end, we will see a commoditisation of basic tracking: Your phone, your earbud, and your thermostat will all track your sleep for free (or for the cost of your data). It will be ubiquitous and low-fidelity. At the top end, we will see the emergence of clinical-grade sleep systems. These will be expensive, subscription-based ecosystems involving smart mattresses, neuro-modulation headbands, and AI coaching. They will be marketed as performance enhancers for the elite and medical necessities for the sick.

The sleep economy is maturing. It is moving from the gadget phase to the infrastructure phase. And as the venture capital flows, it is rewriting the social contract of the night: sleep is no longer a free natural resource; it is a complex asset class to be managed, optimised, and ultimately, sold.

12

The Future of Sleep

> A good laugh and a long sleep are the best cures in the doctor's book.

IRISH PROVERB

The End of the Beginning

We began this journey with the story of Myra Juliet Farrell, the remarkable woman who invented the stitchless button in her sleep. Back in 1915, she understood instinctively what modern science is only just beginning to confirm in the late 2020s. She knew that the night is not a dead zone or a waste of time; it is a workshop. Myra did not need a smart ring, a neural headband, or a haptic mattress to innovate. She simply needed to trust her own biology. She viewed sleep not as a tax on her time but as a vital tool for her mind.

Somewhere along the way, modern society lost that trust. We spent the better part of the twentieth century waging a war on the night. We enlisted the electric light bulb to banish the dark and used the industrial clock to colonise our circadian rhythms. We treated rest as a weakness, a biological flaw to be minimised in the relentless pursuit of productivity. When our bodies inevitably broke under the strain, we tried to fix them with chemical hammers. We used sedatives to knock us out and stimulants to wake us up rather than repairing the foundation of our health.

Now, we stand at the threshold of a new era. We have moved from the industrial age of sleep to the information age of sleep. The 'Internet of Bodies' has turned the average bedroom into a decentralised clinical lab. Artificial Intelligence is evolving from a passive tracker into an active co-pilot. The 'Programmable Sanctuary' is no longer science fiction, it is a reality where the very air and light of our rooms are engineered to induce recovery.

This is the future of sleep. Yet technology is merely the vehicle, it is not the destination. The ultimate goal of all this high-fidelity sensing and algorithmic coaching is not to become dependent on machines. It is to use the machines to relearn how to be human.

The Death of the Passive Tracker

If the last decade was defined by the question *How well did I sleep?*, the next decade will be defined by the answer *Here is ex-*

actly how you can sleep better. We are witnessing the death of the passive tracker and the rise of the active intervention.

The era of the quantified self is coming to an end. For too long, we have obsessively collected data we did not know how to use. We have stared at red scores on our phones and felt a pang of guilt or anxiety known as orthosomnia without having any clear path to improvement. We were drowning in data but starving for solutions.

We are now entering the era of the automated environment: The future bedroom will be a closed-loop system that operates without your constant input. You will not need to look at a sleep score in the morning to know you were hot. Your mattress will have already cooled you down at 3am because it detected a spike in your heart rate. You will not need to remember to dim the lights. Your home automation system, synced to your circadian digital twin, will have shifted the spectrum to amber before you even finished dinner.

This shift from monitoring to modulation is profound. It moves the heavy burden of sleep hygiene from the user to the infrastructure. It acknowledges that willpower is a finite resource, especially when we are tired. By offloading the logistics of the night to an AI agent, or our sleep concierge/team, we free up the cognitive space to actually relax. We are moving from a model where we serve the technology by logging, tagging, and syncing to a model where the technology finally serves us.

The Great Convergence: Biology and Business

The boundaries between the hospital and the home have dissolved. The consumerisation of #MedTech means that the device on your wrist is no longer just a pedometer. It is a diagnostic tool capable of detecting sleep apnoea, atrial fibrillation, and the early signs of infection. This convergence is a double-edged sword. On one hand, it democratises health in a way we have never seen before. It allows for the early detection of conditions that would otherwise go undiagnosed for years. It puts the power of the sleep lab directly into the hands of the patient, and this empowers individuals to take control of their health destiny. On the other hand, it creates the medical-consumer blurring of lines. We risk pathologising normal life by turning every dip in deep sleep into a symptom and every restless night into a medical event. We are creating a class of the worried well who are digitally anxious about metrics that may not even be perfectly accurate.

The business of sleep is betting big that you will pay for peace of mind. We are moving from a transactional economy, where you might buy a bed once every ten years, to a subscription economy. Sleep is becoming SaaS (Software as a Service). You will rent your comfort, you will subscribe to your temperature control. Your ability to rest is becoming a line item on your monthly credit card statement, sitting right next to your internet bill and your streaming services.

The Bifurcation of Rest

As we look toward 2040, a shadow looms over the sleep land-scape. This is the risk of inequality. We are seeing a bifurcation of good sleep where access to rest depends heavily on socioeconomic status. At the top end, the sleep elite will have access to digital twins that simulate their jet lag protocols. They will have mattresses that actively regulate their core temperature and neuro-modulation devices that zap their vagus nerves into serenity. They will use sleep as a performance-enhancing drug to widen the gap in health, longevity, and economic productivity. They will check into 'Sleep Tourism' retreats to repair their circadian rhythms and use dream engineering to boost their creativity. At the bottom end, the precariat and proletariat will continue to suffer from noise pollution, shift work disorder, and the heat island effect of warming cities. Their sleep data may be harvested not to help them but to judge them. Employers might use it to monitor readiness, or insurers might use it to adjust premiums based on risk.

This is why the future of sleep is political. It is not enough to build better gadgets. We must build better policies. The 'Right to Disconnect' must evolve from a European labour experiment into a global human right. We must recognise that the gender data gap has left half the population navigating the night with a map drawn for someone else. We must demand that the next generation of tech is #FemTech2.0, which is cycle-aware, biologically inclusive, and designed for the reality of female physiology.

Data Habeas Corpus: Owning the Night

As we invite radar into our bedrooms and allow algorithms to interpret our dreams, we must remain vigilant about the data ecosystem and start to think of it like a map of the London Underground. We have built a glass bedroom that is transparent to data brokers, advertisers, and insurance companies. We need zero-knowledge architectures where the insights are generated locally on your device and the raw data never leaves your possession. We need the right to data portability to allow us to take our sleep history from one platform to another without penalty. We need to reject the walled gardens that try to lock us in by holding our biological history hostage. The sleep agent (read: Mr Smith of the Matrix) of the future must work for you and not for a tech giant, it must be a fiduciary of your health. Fundamentally, it must be bound by a digital Hippocratic Oath to protect your privacy as fiercely as it protects your rest.

The Return to the Cave

Ultimately, the most sophisticated technology discussed in this book is trying to replicate something very primitive. We are using lasers, algorithms, AI, and haptics to rebuild the conditions of the cave. We use pink noise to mimic the wind and rain, we use blackout curtains and melanopic-safe lighting to mimic the setting sun. We use weighted blankets and haptic wearables to mimic the safety of the tribe's embrace. We use targeted memory reactivation to do what storytellers did around the fire for millennia by consolidating wisdom. It is all derivative of an innate *Sapiens* skill or setting.

There is a beautiful irony in this: We are building a technological cocoon to protect us from the technological world we created. We are fighting fire with data and using the most advanced tools humanity has ever invented to achieve the most ancient of human states. The successful sleeper of 2040 will not be the one with the most gadgets strapped to their head. It will be the one who uses technology to remove friction and then knows when to stop. The true sleep co-pilot is one that lands the plane safely and then shuts down the engines.

A Manifesto for the Night

So, how do we navigate this brave new world? How do we become sleep engineers without becoming Orthosomniacs, terrifyingly obsessed with the sleep score? Here are five principles for the new era of sleep:

1. Respect the Biology

You are an ancient organism in a modern cage. Your body runs on a solar clock and a lunar cycle. It is not a machine that can be rebooted at will. It is a biological system that requires rhythm. Use technology to align with these rhythms rather than to override them. Do not use coffee to fight a circadian dip. Use light to shift the clock. Do not use pills to force a shutdown. Use temperature to trigger the onset.

2. Audit Your Environment

Your bedroom is a machine for rest. Is it doing its job? Perform the sensory audit. Tape over the standby LEDs. Seal the light leaks. Filter the air. Control the noise floor. If you wouldn't expect a plant to thrive in a dark and stuffy box, do not expect your brain to thrive in one. The environment dictates the behaviour.

3. Trust Your Feelings, Verify with Data

The device is a compass. It is not a GPS. If your 'Readiness Score' says you are tired but you feel great, trust your body. If the data says you slept well but you feel exhausted, trust your body. Use the data to spot long-term trends and identify invisible disruptors like alcohol or late meals. Live in the immediate sensation of your own energy. Do not outsource your interoception to a silicon chip.

4. Protect Your Privacy

Your sleep is your most vulnerable state. Treat the data you generate with the same caution you treat your financial records. Choose platforms that encrypt data. Reject services that sell anonymised insights to third parties. Demand interoperability. If you cannot export your data in a readable format, you do not own it, you are just renting it.

5. Reframe Rest

Sleep is not the absence of work. It is the foundation of it. It is logistics. It is the supply chain of your cognitive capital. Treat it with the same professional rigour you treat your bank account or your calendar. In a world of burnout, the sleepless elite are dinosaurs. The future belongs to the well-rested leaders who have the emotional resilience and cognitive clarity to navigate complexity.

Final Thoughts

We are living through a revolution. The 'black box' of sleep has been opened, just like Pandora's, and we can now see all the gears turning. We can watch the dance of the neurons, the flush of the glymphatic system, and the rhythm of the hormones. But with this visibility comes responsibility; we must choose how we use this power. We can use it to turn ourselves into optimised robots that squeeze every drop of productivity out of our resting hours. Or we can use it to reclaim our humanity. We can use the sleep economy to buy back the silence we lost. We can use the internet of bodies to understand the whispers of our own physiology. We can use dream engineering not to sell products but to solve problems and heal trauma.

The future of sleep is bright because it is finally yours to control. We have the tools, the science, and the understanding to banish the exhausted century and usher in an age of restoration. The night belongs to you. It is your workshop, your sanctuary, and your second shift.

So, turn off the light, close your eyes, and let the engineering begin.

Sleep well and Beaux Rêves.

Acknowledgements

To my bed, my ergonomic bamboo pillow, and my air conditioning. Thank you.

I mostly wrote this book listening to the 'focus' music in the Headspace app, which I paid for. It really helped.

Have to say I didn't get great sleep whilst finishing this book thanks to 2 boys under 8. In fact, I haven't had a good night's sleep for 9 years, really. I am starting to have hope I could make a night through uninterrupted if I just got myself to a place with double glazing, noise reduction, and no one needing me in the middle of the night.

Always thanks to you, J, for helping me carry the load. What a man, what a mighty good man.

Directory of Sleep Technology

<u>Hardware & Wearables (The Quantified Self)</u>

Apple Watch: www.apple.com — Mainstream wearable with FDA-cleared AFib and Sleep Apnoea detection features.

Circular: circular.xyz — Smart ring with vibration feedback for silent alarms and bio-signal tracking.

Evie Ring (Movano Health): eviering.com — The first smart ring designed specifically for women's health, tracking sleep, activity, and menstrual cycles with medical-grade sensors.

Fitbit (Google): fitbit.com — Activity trackers with "Sleep Profile" and stress management analysis.

Frenz Brainband (Earable Neuroscience): frenzband.com — An AI-powered headband that uses bone-conduction audio and real-time brainwave monitoring to induce sleep and focus.

Garmin: garmin.com — Performance watches featuring "Body Battery" energy monitoring and advanced sleep staging.

Google Nest Hub: store.google.com — Bedside device using "Soli" radar for contactless sleep sensing.

Oura Ring: ouraring.com — The market-leading smart ring for sleep staging and readiness tracking.

Samsung Galaxy Watch / Ring: samsung.com — Smartwatches and the Galaxy Ring featuring "Energy Score" and sleep apnea detection.

Sleepal AI Lamp (XSmart Century Technology): sleepal.ai — A contact-free sleep tracking lamp (CES 2026 Honoree) that uses millimeter-wave radar to monitor sleep and environmental quality without cameras.

Ultrahuman: ultrahuman.com — Metabolic health-focused smart ring (Ring Air) and the "Ultrahuman Home" environment monitor.

Whoop: whoop.com — Subscription-based recovery strap focusing on strain and HRV.

Withings: withings.com — Makers of the "ScanWatch" and "Sleep Analyzer" under-mattress mats.

Neuro-Modulation & Bio-Hacking (The Switches for Calm)

Apollo Neuro: apolloneuro.com — Wrist/ankle wearable that uses "touch therapy" (haptic vibrations) to balance the nervous system.

Dodow: various sleep retailers in your country — Light-based metronome for breathing entrainment and sleep induction.

Dormio: media.mit.edu — The MIT Media Lab project for Targeted Dream Incubation (TDI).

Dreem (Beacon Biosignals): beacon.bio — Clinical-grade EEG headbands (now primarily focused on research/pharma markets).

Elemind: elemindtech.com — A neuro-stimulation headband that actively cancels out "wake" brainwaves to induce sleep faster.

Embr Wave: embrlabs.com — Wrist-worn thermal regulation device ("Personal Thermostat") for hot flashes and comfort.

Hapbee: hapbee.com — Wearable using magnetic field technology to mimic chemical states (alertness/sleep).

Moonbird: moonbird.life — A handheld, tactile breathing coach that expands and contracts to guide slow-paced breathing for anxiety reduction.

Muse: choosemuse.com — EEG headband for meditation feedback and sleep support ("Digital Sleeping Pill").

Nurosym (Parasym): nurosym.com — Earpiece for transcutaneous auricular vagus nerve stimulation (taVNS).

Ozlo Sleepbuds: ozlosleep.com — The successors to Bose Sleepbuds; tiny, masking earbuds with biometric sensors for sleep.

Pulsetto: pulsetto.tech — Vagus nerve stimulator worn around the neck for rapid stress reduction.

Sensate: getsensate.com— Chest-worn device using infra-sonic resonance to tone the vagus nerve.

Somnee: somneesleep.com — A smart headband that uses non-invasive brain stimulation (tES) to improve sleep duration and quality.

WillSleep (NeuroTx): neurotx.kr — A wearable patch presented at CES 2026 for transcutaneous vagus nerve stimulation (nVNS) to treat insomnia.

Sleep Environment & The Programmable Sanctuary

10minds (Motion Pillow): 10minds.com — An AI-powered pillow that detects snoring and inflates internal airbags to gently turn the user's head.

ANSSil (SomaNest & OptimizeME): anssil.com — A smart air-mattress system (CES 2026 Honoree) that uses "Sync AI" to adjust firmness and angle in real-time based on sleep stages.

BedJet: bedjet.com — Air-based rapid cooling and heating system for beds.

Bryte: bryte.com — AI-powered restorative mattress often found in luxury hotels.

Casper: casper.com — Direct-to-consumer mattresses and "Glow" sleep lights.

Ceragem (Neuro Wellness Youth Bed): ceragem.com — A smart bed designed for adolescents (CES 2026 Innovation Award) featuring spinal thermal massage and an AI health concierge.

ChiliSleep (Sleepme): sleep.me — Water-based cooling pads ("Dock Pro" / "OOLER") for precise temperature control.

DeRucci: global.derucci.com — Makers of the "T11 Pro" AI mattress series which includes 23 sensors to track position, temperature, and heart rate to auto-adjust firmness.

Dyson: dyson.com — Air purifiers for allergen and particulate matter filtration.

Eight Sleep: eightsleep.com — "The Pod" smart mattress cover with active heating/cooling and biometric tracking (Pod 4/5 Ultra).

ERA Smart Layer (Welltech Electronics): eraadaptiveintelligence.com — A smart mattress topper (CES 2025 Honoree) that adds active spinal alignment and BCG sensing to any standard bed.

ErgoSportive (Ergomotion): ergosportive.com — A smart adjustable bed base with sensors that integrate directly with Garmin wearables for recovery tracking.

Ergomotion (RIO Eco): ergomotion.com — A sustainable smart bed base (CES 2026) made from recycled materials, featuring the "Sleep Assist" app for snore intervention and zero-gravity presets.

Hästens: hastens.com — Ultra-luxury natural material beds (The "Vividus").

LG Electronics (Smart Bed): lg.com — Presented "Affectionate Intelligence" at CES 2025, a smart bed hub that controls room humidity and temperature based on health data like coughing.

mui Lab: muilab.com — Creators of the "mui Board" and "Calm Sleep Platform," a wood-based spatial AI interface that tracks sleep without cameras or wearables.

Netatmo: netatmo.com — Smart home weather stations monitoring Indoor CO2, noise, and temperature.

Philips Hue: philips-hue.com — Smart lighting for circadian control (amber/red light scenes).

Purple: purple.com — Gel-grid mattresses for pressure relief and airflow.

Simba: simbasleep.com — Hybrid mattresses using titanium springs and foam.

Sleep Number: sleepnumber.com — Adjustable firmness smart beds with "SleepIQ" technology and new "next-gen" features announced for 2026.

Tempur-Pedic: tempurpedic.com — "TEMPUR-Ergo" smart bases with snore detection and vibration response.

Women's Sleep Tech & Menopause (Femtech)

Dagsmejan: dagsmejan.com — Temperature-regulating sleepwear using lyocell and merino blends.

Femography: femography.com — Advanced apparel technology for menopausal health including the brand 'Become'.

Natural Cycles: naturalcycles.com — Thermometer-based app (often paired with Oura) for cycle tracking and infradian rhythm awareness.

Terra by Amira: amira.care — A predictive cooling mattress pad designed specifically to detect and neutralise hot flashes before they wake you.

Medical Devices & Therapeutics (Rx & Clinical Grade)

Bongo Rx: bongorx.com — Expiratory Positive Airway Pressure (EPAP) nasal valves.

eXciteOSA: exciteosa.com — Daytime therapy device to strengthen tongue muscles and reduce snoring.

Inspire Medical Systems: inspiresleep.com — Implantable hypoglossal nerve stimulation for sleep apnoea (The "Pacemaker for the tongue").

NightWare: nightware.com — Prescription digital therapeutic (Apple Watch app) for PTSD-related nightmares.

Philips Respironics: Philips.com — CPAP and home ventilation solutions.

Remedē System (Respicardia): respicardia.com — Implantable system for Central Sleep Apnea.

ResMed: resmed.com — Global leader in cloud-connected CPAP machines (AirSense 11).

SomnoMed: somnomed.com — Custom-made oral appliances (mandibular advancement devices).

WatchPAT (Itamar Medical): zoll.com — The standard for home sleep apnea testing (HSAT) using finger-based biosensors.

Wesper: wesper.co — FDA-cleared at-home sleep apnoea testing patches that provide clinical-grade diagnostics.

Apps, AI & Digital Services (Software as Medicine)

Calm: calm.com — Meditation, "Sleep Stories," and soundscapes.

Headspace: headspace.com — Mindfulness, "Sleepcasts," and focus tools.

Pzizz: pzizz.com — Psychoacoustic audio for naps and sleep induction.

Rise Science: risescience.com — App focused on sleep debt and circadian energy management.

Sleep Cycle: sleepcycle.com — Smart alarm clock that tracks sleep phases via microphone.

SleepFM (Stanford University): www.stanford.edu — An AI foundation model developed to predict disease risk from sleep data.

Sleepio (Big Health): sleepio.com — Digital Cognitive Behavioural Therapy (dCBTI) for insomnia.

SnoreLab: snorelab.com — Audio recording and analysis app for snoring monitoring.

Somryst: somryst.com — Prescription digital therapeutic for chronic insomnia.

Timeshifter: timeshifter.com — Circadian app for jet lag and shift work (used by astronauts).

Parenting & Infant Sleep (The Fourth Trimester)

CuboAi: cuboai.com — AI baby monitor with face cover detection.

Hatch: hatch.co — Smart sound machines and night lights ("Rest").

Nanit: nanit.com — Computer vision baby monitor with breathing wear tracking.

Owlet: owletcare.com — "Smart Sock" monitoring infant heart rate and oxygen.

Snoo (Happiest Baby): happiestbaby.com — Robotic smart bassinet that responds to crying.

Hospitality & Sleep Tourism

Equinox Hotels: equinox-hotels.com — Performance-focused hotels with soundproofing and cryotherapy.

Hästens Sleep Spa: www.hastens.com/en/hospitality — A hotel in Portugal dedicated to the experience of their mattresses.

Park Hyatt (New York): hyatt.com — Features "Restorative Sleep Suites" with Bryte beds.

Six Senses: sixsenses.com — Luxury resorts with dedicated "Sleep with Six Senses" clinical programs.

AI Declaration

A Note on Artificial Intelligence

While this book explores the future of technology, the vision, stories, and ideas within it are distinctly human and entirely my own.

In the spirit of the "active co-pilot" discussed in these pages, I utilised ChatGPT Pro and Gemini Pro as my digital research assistants. They served as tireless librarians, fact-checkers, and reference finders. Most importantly, they were always available for a chat at 3am and really good at helping me refine my thinking when the rest of the world was fast asleep.

I also had to fact check and double reference check every recommendation because of AIs still having 'hallucinations' in 2026... and I caught a few, naughty AIs.

References and Further Reading

Akerstedt, T., & Wright, K. P. (2009). Sleep loss and fatigue in shift work and shift work disorder. *Sleep Medicine Clinics*, 4(2), 257-271

Ball, C., (2022) *Converge: A futurist's insights into the potential of our world as technology and humanity collide. (Major St Publishing)* www.drcatherineball.com

Baker, F. C., & Driver, H. S. (2007). Circadian rhythms, sleep, and the menstrual cycle. *Sleep Medicine*, 8(6), 613-622.

Baron, K. G., et al. (2017). Orthosomnia: Are some patients taking the quantified self too far? *Journal of Clinical Sleep Medicine*, 13(2), 351-354.

Besedovsky, L., Lange, T., & Born, J. (2019). The sleep-immune crosstalk in health and disease. *Physiological Reviews*, 99(3), 1325-1380.

Biswas, A. (2025). *Building agentic AI systems.*

Blume, C., Garbazza, C., & Spitschan, M. (2019). Effects of light on human circadian rhythms, sleep and mood. *Somnologie*, 23(3), 147-156.

Bonafide CP, Localio AR, Ferro DF, et al. Accuracy of Pulse Oximetry-Based Home Baby Monitors. JAMA. 2018;320(7):717–719.

Buysse, D. J. (2013). Insomnia. *JAMA*, 309(7), 706-716.

Cajochen, C., et al. (2011). Evening exposure to a light-emitting diodes (LED)-backlit computer screen affects circadian physiology and cognitive performance. *Journal of Applied Physiology*, 110(5), 1432-1438.

A. Chang, D. Aeschbach, J.F. Duffy, & C.A. Czeisler, (2015). Evening use of light-emitting eReaders negatively affects sleep, circadian timing, and next-morning alertness, Proc. Natl. Acad. Sci. U.S.A. 112 (4) 1232-1237,

Cohen, S., Doyle, W. J., Alper, C. M., Janicki-Deverts, D., & Turner, R. B. (2009). Sleep habits and susceptibility to the common cold. *Archives of Internal Medicine*, 169(1), 62-67.

Dijk D-J, Archer SN (2009) Light, Sleep, and Circadian Rhythms: Together Again. PLoS Biol 7(6): e1000145.

Dolev, Z. (2019). Sleep and Women's Health. (1st ed.). CRC Press LLC.

Dubief, A. (2018). *Precious little sleep*. https://www.precious-littlesleep.com

Gottfried, S. (2013). *The hormone cure*. Scribner. https://www.saragottfriedmd.com

Gunter, J. (2021). *The menopause manifesto*. Citadel Press. https://drjengunter.com

Harari, Y. N. (2024). *Nexus: A brief history of information networks from the Stone Age to AI*. Fern Press. https://www.ynharari.com

Herring, W. J., Connor, K. M., Ivgy-May, N., Snyder, E., Liu, K., Snavely, D. B., Krystal, A. D., Walsh, J. K., Benca, R. M., Rosenberg, R., Sangal, R. B., Budd, K., Hutzelmann, J., Leibensperger, H., Froman, S., Lines, C., Roth, T., & Michelson, D. (2016). Suvorexant in Patients With Insomnia: Results From Two 3-Month Randomized Controlled Clinical Trials. *Biological psychiatry*, *79*(2), 136–148.

Huyen, C. (2025). *AI engineering*. https://huyenchip.com

Iliff, J. J., et al. (2012). A paravascular pathway facilitates CSF flow through the brain parenchyma and the clearance of interstitial solutes, including amyloid β. *Science Translational Medicine*, 4(147), 147ra111.

Karp H. (2012). The fourth trimester and the calming reflex: novel ideas for nurturing young infants. *Midwifery today with international midwife*, (102), 25–67.

Karp, H. (2002). *The happiest baby on the block*. Bantam. https://www.happiestbaby.com

Krause, A. J., Prather, A. A., Wager, T. D., Lindquist, M. A., & Walker, M. P. (2019). The Pain of Sleep Loss: A Brain Characterization in Humans. *The Journal of neuroscience : the official journal of the Society for Neuroscience*, *39*(12), 2291–2300.

Kryger, M. H. (2017). The mystery of sleep: why a good night's rest is vital to a better, healthier life (First edition.). Yale University Press.

Kurzweil, R. (2024). *The singularity is nearer: When we merge with AI*. Viking.

Lloyd-Jones, D. M., et al. (2022). Life's essential 8: Updating and enhancing the American Heart Association's construct of cardiovascular health. *Circulation*, 146(5), e18-e43.

Mallampalli, M. P., & Carter, C. L. (2014). Exploring sex and gender differences in sleep health: A Society for Women's Health Research report. *Journal of Women's Health*, 23(7), 553-562.

McGraw, K., et al. (1999). Development of circadian rhythms of self-selected sleep and activity in full-term infants. *Sleep*, 22(3), 303-310.

McGregor, A. (2020). *Sex matters: How male-centric medicine endangers women's health*. Hachette Books.

McKenna, J. J. (2020). *Safe infant sleep: Expert answers to your cosleeping questions*. Platypus Media.

Medina, J. (2014). *Brain rules for baby*. Pear Press.

Monteleone, P., Mascagni, G., Giannini, A., Genazzani, A. R., & Simoncini, T. (2018). Symptoms of menopause - global trends in etiology, prevalence and management. *Nature Reviews Endocrinology*, 14, 199-215.

Moon, R. Y., et al. (2022). Sleep-related infant deaths: Updated 2022 recommendations for a safe infant sleeping environment. *Pediatrics*, 150(1).

Nedergaard, M., & Goldman, S. A. (2020). Glymphatic failure as a final common pathway to dementia. *Science*, 370(6512), 50-56.

Nestor, J. (2020). *Breath: The new science of a lost art*. Riverhead Books.

Okun M. L. (2015). Sleep and postpartum depression. *Current opinion in psychiatry*, 28(6), 490–496.

Panda, S. (2018). *The circadian code*. Rodale Books.

Pantley, E. (2002). *The no-cry sleep solution*. McGraw-Hill.

Polo-Kantola, P. (2011). Sleep problems in midlife and beyond. Maturitas, 68(3), 224–232.

Prather, A. A., Janicki-Deverts, D., Hall, M. H., & Cohen, S. (2015). Behaviorally assessed sleep and susceptibility to the common cold. *Sleep*, 38(9), 1353-1359.

Rasch, B., & Born, J. (2013). About sleep's role in memory. *Physiological Reviews*, 93(2), 681-766.

Richter, D., et al. (2019). Long-term effects of pregnancy and childbirth on sleep satisfaction and duration of first-time and experienced mothers and fathers. *Sleep*, 42(4).

Saper, C. B., Scammell, T. E., & Lu, J. (2005). The sleep switch: Hypothalamic control of sleep and wakefulness. *Trends in Neurosciences*, 28(12), 710-716.

Spiegel, K., Leproult, R., & Van Cauter, E. (1999). Impact of sleep debt on metabolic and endocrine function. *Lancet (London, England)*, *354*(9188), 1435–1439.

Subasi, A. (Ed.). (2025). *Artificial intelligence applications for brain-computer interfaces*.

Tononi, G., & Cirelli, C. (2014). Sleep and the price of plasticity: From synaptic and cellular homeostasis to memory consolidation and integration. *Neuron*, 81(1), 12-34.

Topol, E. (2019). *Deep medicine: How artificial intelligence can make healthcare human again*. Basic Books.

Vitti, A. (2020). *In the FLO*. HarperOne.

Walker, M. P. (2009). The role of sleep in cognition and emotion. *Annals of the New York Academy of Sciences*, 1156(1), 168-197.

Walker, M. (2017). *Why we sleep: Unlocking the power of sleep and dreams*. Scribner.

Wickramasinghe, N. (2025). *Digital twins: For superior clinical decision making*.

Winter, W. C. (2017). *The sleep solution: Why your sleep is broken and how to fix it*. Berkley.

Wolpaw, J. R., & Wolpaw, E. W. (Eds.). (2012). *Brain-computer interfaces: Principles and practice*. Oxford University Press.

Wu, J. (2023). *Hello sleep: The science and art of overcoming insomnia without medications*. St. Martin's Press.

Xie, L., et al. (2013). Sleep drives metabolite clearance from the adult brain. *Science, 342*(6156), 373-377.

Zuboff, S. (2019). *The age of surveillance capitalism: The fight for a human future at the new frontier of power*. PublicAffairs.

Acronyms and Abbreviations

A–D

- **AAP**: American Academy of Pediatrics
- **AFib**: Atrial Fibrillation
- **AHI**: Apnoea-Hypopnoea Index
- **AI**: Artificial Intelligence
- **API**: Application Programming Interface
- **ARR**: Annual Recurring Revenue
- **AWS**: Amazon Web Services
- **BCI**: Brain-Computer Interface
- **BLE**: Bluetooth Low Energy
- **BMI**: Body Mass Index
- **CBTI / dCBTI**: Cognitive Behavioural Therapy for Insomnia (Digital)
- **CCPA**: California Consumer Privacy Act
- **CES**: Consumer Electronics Show
- **CO2**: Carbon Dioxide
- **COPD**: Chronic Obstructive Pulmonary Disease
- **CPAP**: Continuous Positive Airway Pressure
- **CSV**: Comma-Separated Values
- **DAO**: Decentralised Autonomous Organisation
- **DiGA**: Digital Health Applications (Germany)
- **DLMO**: Dim Light Melatonin Onset
- **DORA**: Dual Orexin Receptor Antagonist
- **DPS**: Deep Pressure Stimulation

- **DTC**: Direct-to-Consumer
- **DTx**: Digital Therapeutics

E–H

- **ECG**: Electrocardiogram
- **EDI**: Equivalent Daylight Illuminance (Melanopic)
- **EEG**: Electroencephalography (Brain waves)
- **EMA**: European Medicines Agency
- **EMG**: Electromyography (Muscle tone)
- **EOG**: Electrooculography (Eye movements)
- **EPAP**: Expiratory Positive Airway Pressure
- **FDA**: Food and Drug Administration
- **FHIR**: Fast Healthcare Interoperability Resources
- **FRMS**: Fatigue Risk Management Systems
- **GABA**: Gamma-Aminobutyric Acid
- **GDPR**: General Data Protection Regulation
- **GLP-1**: Glucagon-like Peptide-1
- **GP**: General Practitioner
- **HCI**: Human-Computer Interaction
- **HEPA**: High Efficiency Particulate Air
- **HIPAA**: Health Insurance Portability and Accountability Act
- **HRT**: Hormone Replacement Therapy
- **HRV**: Heart Rate Variability
- **HSAT**: Home Sleep Apnoea Test
- **HSE**: Health and Safety Executive
- **HVAC**: Heating, Ventilation, and Air Conditioning

I–P

- **ICU**: Intensive Care Unit
- **IoB**: Internet of Bodies
- **ipRGCs**: Intrinsically Photosensitive Retinal Ganglion Cells
- **IRT**: Imagery Rehearsal Therapy
- **JSON**: JavaScript Object Notation
- **LD**: Lucid Dreaming
- **LED**: Light Emitting Diode
- **LLM**: Large Language Model
- **MSLT**: Multiple Sleep Latency Test
- **NASA**: National Aeronautics and Space Administration
- **NREM**: Non-Rapid Eye Movement
- **OSA**: Obstructive Sleep Apnoea
- **PCM**: Phase Change Materials
- **PCOS**: Polycystic Ovary Syndrome
- **PDF**: Portable Document Format
- **PhD**: Doctor of Philosophy
- **PPG**: Photoplethysmography
- **ppm**: Parts per million
- **PSG**: Polysomnogram
- **PTSD**: Post-Traumatic Stress Disorder

R–Z

- **RBD**: REM Sleep Behaviour Disorder
- **REM**: Rapid Eye Movement
- **RPM**: Remote Patient Monitoring
- **SaaS**: Sleep-as-a-Service
- **SaMD**: Software as a Medical Device

- **SRT**: Sleep Restriction Therapy
- **SSI**: Self-Sovereign Identity
- **tACS**: Transcranial Alternating Current Stimulation
- **taVNS**: Transcutaneous Auricular Vagus Nerve Stimulation
- **TDI**: Targeted Dream Incubation
- **TGA**: Therapeutic Goods Administration
- **TMR**: Targeted Memory Reactivation
- **VC**: Venture Capital
- **VMS**: Vasomotor Symptom
- **VNS**: Vagus Nerve Stimulation
- **VR**: Virtual Reality
- **YASA**: Yet Another Spindle Algorithm